Copper: Quest for a Cure

John Walshe, MD, ScD, FRCP.

Emeritus Reader in Metabolic Disease, University of Cambridge

Formerly Honorary Consultant Physician, Addenbrooke's Hospital, Cambridge
and
The Middlesex Hospital, London

ACKNOWLEDGEMENTS

I wish to thank the following copyright holders for permission to publish the following illustrations. The Editor of Brain and the Oxford University Press for permission to publish plates 2 and 5 which appeared in Brain, 2009, 132, 2289-2295. (The Conquest of Wilson's Disease, J.M.Walshe) Also the Editor of Movement Disorders Journal and John Wiley and Sons, Inc. for permission to publish figure 4 which appeared as fart of figure 8 in Movement Disorders, 1999, 14, 545-550, (J.M.Walshe, Penicillamine, Treatment of choice for patients with Wilson's Disease). Also Figures 1,8 and 9 which appeared in Movement disorders, 2003, 18, 853-859 (J.M.Walshe, The Story of Penicillamine: a difficult Birth).

TABLE OF CONTENTS

FOREWORD

Dr John Walshe's contribution to patients with Wilson's disease is perhaps a unique example in clinical medicine where one individual has been fundamental in the treatment and survival of patients and where a lifelong interest and commitment to such a group has achieved so much.

Early in his career, in the early 1950s, John Walshe worked in the metabolic unit at University College Hospital, London, with Dr Charles Dent. Later, while on a fellowship at Boston City Hospital, Massachusetts, it was a stroke of genius (he calls it 'inspiration') that led him to suggest that a urinary metabolite he had identified at UCL could be used orally as a copper chelator for a patient with Wilson's disease. As a result of this insight, D-penicillamine was introduced in 1956 to treat patients with Wilson's disease. Their previous clinical progression to death was reversed and the majority were able to survive with treatment. This was a lifesaving innovation and owes everything not only to the initial recognition of this form of treatment but also to Dr Walshe's tenacity and drive to optimise the treatment of patients with Wilson's disease in the UK and throughout the world.

In this biography Dr Walshe describes events leading up to his discovery of D-penicillamine, obstacles which he had to overcome, the development of other orally-administered drugs to treat Wilson's disease, and his personal care to patients with this rare condition, which few clinicians will have encountered in their careers. This book is a fascinating insight of basic and clinical research in the medical schools and universities of the 1950s, 60s and 70s. It documents both the rewards and also the difficulties of Clinical and Academic Medicine.

This account will be of interest to all who are or have been involved with patients who have Wilson's disease, as well as students of the history of medicine, particularly of clinical academic work through this extraordinary period of intellectual freedom. Such freedom blossomed in the mid 1940s; the ethos continued in subsequent decades and does so today but with often more restraints.

Dr John Walshe deserves our deepest gratitude for all his contributions to patients with Wilson's disease, and for giving us this fascinating account of his life's work.

James Dooley
Consultant Physician Royal Free Hospital
London

PREFACE

I have a tale to tell. Tell me your tale oh.
Gilbert and Sullivan, Yeoman of the Guard.

This is the story of how medical research was carried out in the second half of the last century. It has never been my habit to keep a diary, except during a couple of years when, as a regimental medical officer in the Middle East theatre, I helped to support a tottering Empire. So I have had to rely on my memory and for any lapses there of, I apologise. When in doubt I have referred back to my list of publications and this has helped to keep things in chronological order. This type of research, which I have here described, is unlikely to be repeated. Now is the era of the big battalions, the big projects and the big budgets. In the spring of 1955 I was working as a postgraduate student in the USA when I saw a patient dying of a rare and invariably fatal disease. I had an idea which I thought, on theoretical grounds, should result in a cure. This is the story of how I spent the next ten years in proving my hypothesis and the subsequent forty years seeking additional treatments and establishing an international centre for the treatment of patients with this condition and in elucidating a better understanding of the mechanisms of the disease. When this project was started there were no ethical committees to monitor and restrict the exploitation of new ideas. The atmosphere surrounding medicine was not litigious and research was encouraged and esteemed. This state of affairs, unhappily, no longer exists in this country. I have little doubt that what I did 50 years ago would not be possible today. Some may think this book is nothing more than a shameless ego trip. I suppose to some extent it is but I would like to think it is more. It is a call to a better understanding of how research is carried out and what rewards, to patient care, it can bring, even when carried out as a one man band, if it is pursued with integrity and determination. In 1982 Dr F.E.Karch edited and published a book, to which I contributed, called 'Orphan Drugs'. In this seven authors described their varying successes in finding, in the words of a review in ' The Lancet,' ***Homes for their orphans…..The tales are sagas of frustration; the repeated banging of heads against the brick walls of drug safety regulation, patent law technicalities, health insurance regulations, government buck passing and, above all, stark commercial reality. Fortunately most of the stories had happy endings, but only because of the quite extraordinary tenacity of these men.*** ' I leave it to the reader to judge the success, or otherwise, of my efforts and to decide if they were a reasonable reward for a lifetime's work.

To have achieved what success that I did I owe thanks to many individuals. First to my father who introduced me to the discipline of medicine and the art of criticism of which he was the peerless master: to Professor Charles Dent who introduced me to the mysteries of metabolic disease and helped with my initial faltering steps in this branch of medicine: to Roland Westall who taught me the basics of ion exchange chromatography: to Dr. Charles Davidson who obtained for me the first two grams of penicillamine which made this whole venture possible: to Dr Hal Dixon who suggested the use of triethylenetetramine as a medical chelating agent and who gave invaluable help in its purification for clinical use: to Stuart Laurie, of the de Montfort University, who provided me with ammonium tetrathiomolybdate of high purity for more than ten years at minimum cost and no gain to himself: to Joy Briggs who helped me set up my laboratory methods in Cambridge: to Kay Gibbs who gave unstinting help for nigh on 30 years in setting up and carrying out many of the laboratory tests used in this study and who got to know all my patients and who knew more about Wilson disease than most doctors: to Dr Gerald Stern who invited me to restart my clinic at University College Hospital in London, on my official retirement in 1987; to Professor Andrew Lees who encouraged me to continue the work at the Middlesex Hospital, London and to Dr Godfrey Gillett who took over the care of my patients on my final retirement in the year 2000. I also owe thanks to Rupert Purchase who devised a method of producing purified trientine on a commercial scale and has given valuable advice on the text and help with the stereochemistry of penicillamine. Thanks are also due to all my patients who unfailingly came for the follow up appointments over many years and who willingly put up with the many investigations, most of which must have seen complex and puzzling, though I hope not too painful, with out a murmur of complaint. Of these I must mention particularly Caroline who set up the Wilson's Disease Support Group and Valerie and Linda who later took over its running. But thanks most of all are due to Ann my wife who put up, uncomplainingly, with my long hours in the laboratory and clinic and my occasional absence at conferences for many years while left with the care of the home and, in the early years, my two daughters. Without her unfailing love and support I could not possibly have carried this project to what I believe came to a successful conclusion.

I hope that the following chapters will make clear some of the difficulties in following a career in clinical research during the second half of the last century. They are much greater today with the problems of Ethical Committees, Government targets, funding problems, the fear of litigation and the danger of falling off the over structured ladder of promotion which has become such a feature of the medical profession at the present time. Research is not a feather bedded occupation for those in ivory towers. It is a hard slog with an uncertain outcome; even the best ideas may come to nought. In my own experience I found that even those which seemed sound theoretically, could prove disappointing. But it is an exciting intellectual challenge and I, for one, would not have wished to have followed a different career.

John Walshe,
University of Cambridge
UK

CHAPTER 1

The Birth of an Idea

'Where shall I begin, please your majesty ?'
'Begin at the beginning', the King said, gravely, 'and go on until you come to the end: then
stop'.
Lewis Carroll, Alice in Wonderland.

Abstract: The story began in 1912, but my involvement only began in 1951. In 1912 Dr Kinnier Wilson, working at the National Hospital for Nervous Diseases in London described a new illness affecting youngsters, the principal symptoms being loss of control of movement and contractures of the limbs. This was always associated with scarring of the liver. All these patients died with in a few months of diagnosis.

Dr Wilson's life long ambition was to find a cure for this disease which became known as Wilson's disease, technically hepatolenticular degeneration.. In 1948 Professor John Cumings, working at the same hospital, showed that patients dying of Wilson's disease all had large abnormal amounts of copper deposited in the brain and in the liver. He suggested that the new metal binding drug, British Antilewisite (BAL) might be used to arrest the course of the disease.

In 1951, working in the Metabolic Unit at University College Hospital in London I discovered that patients treated with the antibiotic penicillin excreted in their urine, a breakdown product of the drug, penicillamine. Later, when studying as a Fulbright Fellow in the Liver Unit at the Boston City Hospital, I saw a patient with Wilson's disease being treated, with little, benefit, with BAL. I suggested that penicillamine had the right structural formula to bind copper and promote its excretion and this would be a more effective treatment than BAL and, could be given my mouth and not by painful injection, it would be easier to give over a lifetime.

What admirable advice for those with a story to tell, probably honoured more in the breach than the observance. In practice advice is always easier to give than to follow. Where does my story begin? Was it on the 'bridge' at the Boston City Hospital in May 1955 when I had an idea that it might be possible to treat patients with that hitherto fatal disease, named after its discoverer, Dr Kinnier Wilson.? Was it further back in time when, in 1951, a middle aged man was admitted to University College Hospital with sudden onset of severe, acute abdominal pain due to bleeding from a nodule in his liver – the relevance of this I will describe later, or was it in 1912 when Dr Kinnier Wilson described a 'new disease', under the title *'Progressive lenticular degeneration: a familial nervous disease associated with cirrhosis of the liver'*, in the medical journal Brain, a disease which now bears his name? Or, to come forward in time, was it in 1948 when Professor John Cumings, working at the National Hospital for Nervous Diseases in London reported that Wilson's disease was caused by the accumulation of abnormal amounts of copper in the liver and brains of sufferers from this very rare disease ? Where do I begin ?

The year 1912 seems to be the logical starting point. In that year Dr Kinnier Wilson, the senior resident at The National Hospital for Diseases of the Nervous System at Queen Square in London, described four patients who he saw himself and six others which he traced in hospital records and the medical literature. They were suffering from a hitherto unrecognized disease: the cardinal features being loss of control of the limbs with spasm of muscles leading to bizarre and abnormal postures as a consequence of the destruction of those centres in the brain controlling movement and this was associated with scarring of the liver. Dr Wilson stated that the liver lesion did not contribute to the patients eventual death, though one of his patients actually died of a complication of his liver cirrhosis. He could only guess as to the cause of the disease which, he noted, occurred in families but he could not determine whether this was due to inheritance or a common factor in the environment affecting all siblings in a family. One of his suggestions was that the liver, in these patients actually elaborated a toxin which damaged the brain. Having no definitive idea as to the underlying cause he was in no position to suggest any treatment though it was and remained his lifelong, but unfulfilled, ambition to find one. The disease appeared always to occur in youngsters and invariably ran a fatal course in months or, at most a few years. Subsequent to Wilson's original account the illness was thought, for many years, to be so rare that it was only mentioned, as small print, in specialist text books. Most medical students never heard of it. I certainly did not when training in the 1940s. During the 1920s it was found that Wilson's disease was inherited in a recessive fashion, that is both parents were involved in transmitting the abnormal gene to the offspring and there was also a suggestion that a metal was involved, both silver and copper being suspect, although in fact an Austrian pathologist, Professor Rumpel, way back in 1913, had already fingered copper as the causative agent.

Then, in 1948, came the first of a series of breakthroughs that have transformed our understanding of the disease mechanism and pointed to the possibility of developing an effective treatment. In that year Professor John Cumings, Professor of Clinical Biochemistry at the National Hospital, who had, in the past, served as Dr Wilson's junior, proved that Wilson's disease was caused by accumulation of excess copper in the liver and brains of these patients; he went on to suggest that the progress of the disease might be halted by treating the patients with a drug commonly known as BAL, short for British Antilewisite. The discovery of this drug is in itself is a story which bears repeating. In 1939 it was feared that Hitler's Luftwaffe would attack British cities with the war gas Lewisite and scientists in Oxford started searching for an antidote. Lewisite is an arsenic based compound which gave the clue as to how it might be combated. The team that carried out this search was headed by Professor Sir Rudolph Peters, Professor of Biochemistry in the University. The compound they designed, and which proved successful, was a simple short chain alcohol with two substituted sulphur atoms which enabled it to bind the arsenic in a tight ring converting the metal into a nontoxic compound; a chemical reaction known as chelation: the word chelation being derived from the Greek word for claw. The problem with BAL, from the patient's point of view, was that it has to be given by a painful injection deep in to the buttock and it has many unpleasant side effects, raising the question, is the cure worse than the disease ? Most patients, faced with a certain fatal outcome, had little difficulty in opting for the cure. Professor Cumings observations were enthusiastically followed in the City Hospital, Boston USA, by Professor Denny Brown, in charge of the Harvard Neurological Unit in that hospital. In 1951 he and his associate Dr. Porter reported some success with this treatment at the same time as did Professor Cumings in London. However it soon became apparent that whilst BAL did lead to considerable improvement in these patients each repeated course of the drug produced less and less effect, a phenomenon known as tachyphylaxis, so that this was clearly not the final answer. A year later, in 1952 there was a further major advance. Working independently in New York, two groups or workers, Drs Scheinberg and Gitlin and Drs. Bearn and Kunkel, both noted that the blue copper carrying protein, caeruloplasmin, was absent or deficient in patients with Wilson's disease. This particular protein had originally been isolated and characterized by two Swedish scientists, Drs Holmberg and Laurell.

They had wondered if this protein might be implicated in the pathogenesis of Wilson's disease but, unfortunately for them, the patient their clinical colleagues gave them to study had been miss diagnosed and did not suffer from Wilson disease, as was later discovered.

After demobilization from the Army in 1948 I returned to the Medical Unit at UCH under a rehabilitation scheme, really as a sort of junior registrar, and subsequently as the first Stothert

Research Fellow of the Royal Society. My own interest in Wilson disease arose quite incidentally. I had seen a single patient in 1948, at University College Hospital, (Fig. **1**) who had been treated with BAL with less than impressive results but I had not given the matter further thought. At that time my own particular interest was in the biochemical disturbances in patients with liver failure, a subject at that time sadly neglected. In 1953. I was also using the recently discovered technique of paper chromatography to define abnormalities of amino acid in these patients. This was first introduced into clinical medicine by Dr. Charles Dent. Charles' pioneering work had helped to transform our understanding of metabolic disease and it was to his help and encouragement I owe much. Charles was an outstanding biochemist and his grasp of metabolic disturbances was far ahead of his time. He could argue, convincingly, that black was white and a few days later, equally convincingly, that white was black. One thing he taught me that stood me in good stead was that in any experiment there must be only a single variable; if there are more than this it becomes impossible to interpret the results. It is a pity more researchers to not realize this.

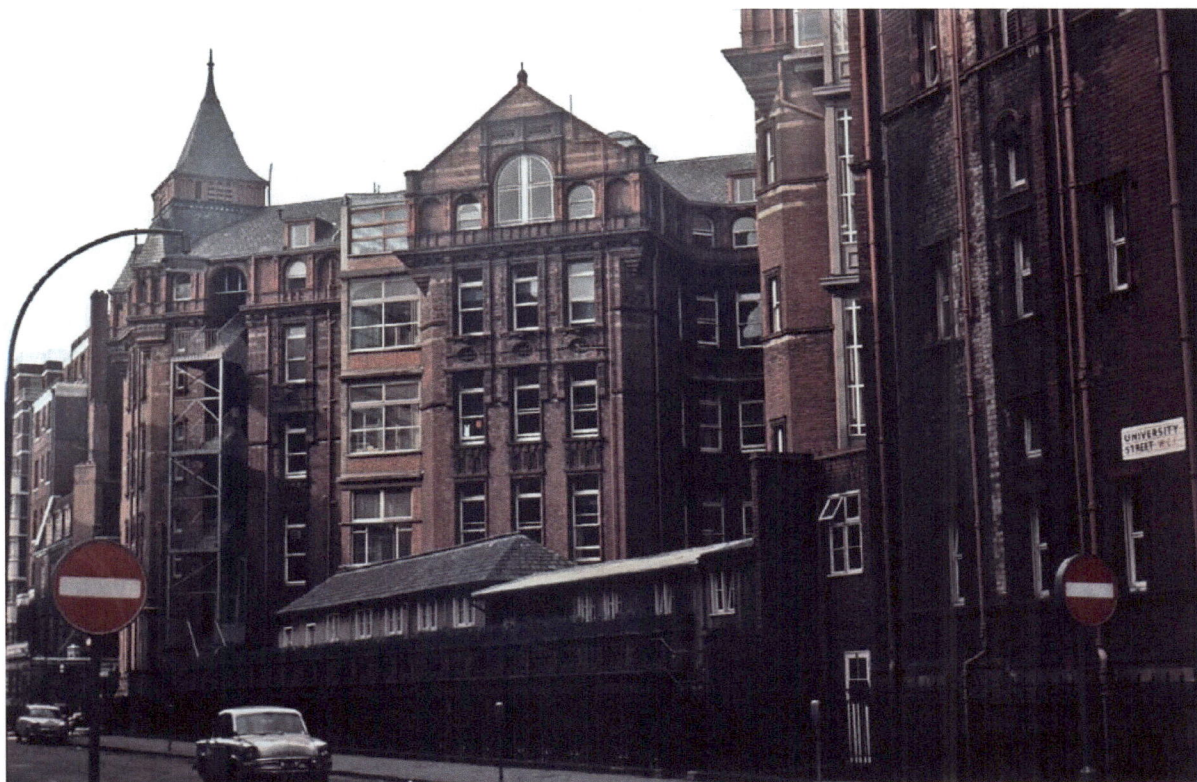

Fig. (1). University College Hospital, the cruciate building, photographed in the early 1950', just after the first appearance of the parking meters in London.

The particular research I was engaged in was studying the pattern of amino acids, the building blocks of protein, which could be identified in blood and urine from patients with liver disease admitted to University College Hospital and comparing these findings with those in the blood and urine of normal people. Some observations led me to introduce the idea of ammonia binding for the treatment of liver coma and I successfully used glutamic acid for this purpose. During the course of this search I was asked to study any possible changes that might occur to the amino acid metabolism of a middle aged man, previously referred to, who was about to have a large section of his liver excised to remove a cancer. After the operation I noted a new unidentified compound appeared in his urine which had never previously been recorded. Using the technique of ion exchange chromatography I was able to isolate and identify this as the amino acid dimethyl cysteine. Charles Dent pointed out to me that this was, in fact a breakdown product of the penicillin, also known as penicillamine. Going back to the patient's notes I realized that this compound only appeared in his urine after his doctors had started treating him with penicillin to combat infection. I then gave myself a large dose of this antibiotic by intravenous injection, the only way penicillin could be administered at that time, and found that I also excreted penicillamine. Further work soon showed that all patients receiving this drug excreted this same compound. This amino acid had originally been described by the Oxford team of Abraham and Chain, Baker and Robinson working with Professor Florey, who were trying to elucidate the structure of penicillin. In their original work they had got the formula wrong as they had mistaken the sulphur atom in the molecule for two atoms of oxygen and this had caused them difficulty in trying to describe the structural formula. This is somewhat surprising as they described how their unknown compound gave a blue colour reaction with ferric chloride which should have alerted them to the presence sulphur in a reactive –SH group. The correct structure of the penicillamine molecule was described later by another Nobel Prize winning chemist Sir John Comforth. His original description was contained in a classified document but was later acknowledged in an article by Harry Crooks, '*Penicillamine its analogs and homologs*'. Penicillamine is an amino acid which can exist in two optically active forms laevo and dextrorotatory depending on the way the amino acid, in solution bends a beam of polarized light. Most such compounds bend light to the left, that they are laevorotatory and are referred to as L- compounds. It so happens that penicillamine produced from penicillin is a D- compound. L-Penicillamine exists and it is the L- form which is produced when penicillamine is syntesissed from other biologically produced amino acids. The distinction is important as L-Penicillamine is toxic being an anntimetabolite for the vitamin pyridoxin, vitamin B6. Patients treated with this form of the compound, as occurred in the United States in the early days, developed loss of vision. The D- form of the compound only has a very weak action in this respect, that is why pyridoxine is given with D-penicillamine under certain very specific circumstances such as pregnancy or during acute illnesses or a growth spurt. From my point of view the finding of penicillamine had proved somewhat disappointing as it did not indicate a new biochemical defect in the patient resulting from surgery to the liver. I included this observation in the MD thesis on amino acid metabolism in liver disease which I submitted to the University of Cambridge but the work was rejected on grounds that it had been included in other published work. I thought this was somewhat harsh and splitting hairs.

The next three years were spent on an entirely different project altogether. I joined up with a young South African doctor, Boris Senior, who had just completed a two year study at the Massachusetts General Hospital in Boston. Under the aegis of Charles Dent we set out to study a condition known as cystinuria, in which cystine stones are formed in the kidneys and bladder. This was believed to be due to an abnormal chemical mechanism in the body which resulted in production of excess of the amino acid cystine. We were able to show that it was in fact due to a defect in kidney function which permitted a leak of the compound into the urine where it crystallized out to form stones. Following this I was awarded a Fulbright Fellowship to the United States to broaden my medical education. In the early 1950's it was virtually a **sine qua non** for any ambitious young doctor to take this step. The initials BTA (Been to America) were almost a higher degree necessary for preferment. Having been awarded the fellowship I needed to find a place of study which would fit my interest and which would be prepared to take me on for a year. At that time the Liver Unit at the Boston City Hospital was one of the leading centres for liver research. This was part of the Harvard Medical Unit at the Hospital under the direction of Dr. Castle (known to his friends as Big Bill Castle) an internationally famous physician for his work on pernicious anaemia. The Liver Unit was directed by Dr. Charles Davidson whose interests were exactly those I wished to pursue. I wrote to him and was at once accepted for the academic year 1954-5. My immediate Professor, Max Rosenheim, director of The Medical Unit at University College Hospital, later to become President of the Royal College of Physicians as Lord Rosenheim, was not too pleased to learn that I had taken this initiative and found acceptance without his advice or approval much less his support; it was simply not the correct procedure to follow. The way was now open for me to return to my primary interest, liver failure and, unbeknownst to me, a new era in my interests was about to open. The next part of my story, and certainly the seminal moment, takes place in the New World.

Thomas Edison once said that '*Genius is one percent inspiration and ninety-nine percent perspiration'*. The next part of my story is of the one percent inspiration. Armed with my Fulbright Fellowship and a position in the Harvard Medical Unit at the Boston City Hospital I set sail for the United States. Way back in 1955 travel was still by sea. In this I was fortunate for my friend and colleague, Dr Freddie Flynn, later to become Professor of Clinical Chemistry at the Middlesex Hospital, London, was also making the journey. We traveled together, sharing a cabin, on the New Amsterdam from Southampton to New York whence he was to go south to Philadelphia whilst I would go north to Boston. The last night of our voyage was enlivened by the passage, up the eastern shores of the US, of hurricane Inez, shades of things to come, the name of my future formidable mother-in–law. This storm somewhat disrupted the rail links that both of us would need to use. In consequence I arrived late in Boston so that my future chief, Dr Charles Davidson (Charlie to his friends), had given up hope of welcoming me and retired home to his apartment overlooking the Charles river. The City Hospital was not situated in the most salubrious part of Boston so my arrival was somewhat daunting. As I made my way from the entrance lobby along endless corridors to the residents quarters, where Dr Davidson had kindly arranged for me to stay, I was somewhat discouraged by the sight of lines of empty jam cans collecting rain water coming through the roof, the legacy of hurricane Inez. The next morning I made my way to the Thorndike Laboratory, where the Liver Unit was established. There I was warmly welcomed by Dr. Davidson, introduced to his team, assigned my place in the laboratory and my assistant for the year, Lee De Carli. Lee was a treasure, very able, hard working and a good friend. I could not have prospered without her help. Badly disabled when young by polio she managed on crutches as if she had almost no disability. Looking around I was not a little surprised to find that the laboratory bench was a trestle table covered with oil cloth, nothing like the chromium plated new world I had led myself to expect. But it did demonstrate that super facilities, though a great help, are not necessary for important advances. It is good ideas that are the vital necessity for real advances in science.

The other graduate members of the team were Les Webster, also working on the biochemistry of liver failure and the biochemist Mike Brinn. Les Webster was full of ideas and always designing the next experiment to prove beyond doubt that the latest idea was correct, always to achieve the opposite result but he never allowed this to discourage him from carrying on the good work. My first task was to find a project which could reasonably be expected to yield some useful results in the course of an academic year. In this quest I was greatly indebted to Mike Brinn who introduced me to a technique for measuring the uptake of oxygen by cells in thin tissue slices, and therefore their metabolic activity. By this method it was possible to investigate the effect of various potentially toxic compounds, which might result from a breakdown of liver function, upon the metabolic activity of the brain. I had been particularly interested in the potential of ammonia to damage brain function, as already mentioned, and had introduced the use of a single amino acid, glutamic acid, to combat this with promising initial results in clinical trials. It was a surprise, therefore, to find that under certain specific circumstances, the brain could itself actually produce and liberate ammonia Thus whilst this work produced a number of interesting results it solved no problems. However, in the spring of the following year, Dr Davidson was invited by Professor Denny Brown to see one of his patients in the Neurology Unit. The patient, who I shall call Joe, was a man in his thirties suffering from Wilson's disease. Joe had been ill for sometime and had been treated with BAL but had not responded particularly well to this treatment. He had a very severe tremor of his arms and trunk and was slipping into liver failure. I wondered how anyone with such a tremor could drive a car safely; perhaps it enabled him to weave his way through the Boston traffic! We were not asked about the management of his Wilson's disease but simply to suggest any treatment which might relieve the problems resulting from his liver damage. On the way back to the Thorndike laboratory, as we were crossing what was known as 'the bridge', an over ground walkway crossing the central courtyard and joining the neurology wards to the Thorndike laboratory (Fig. **2**), I had that moment of inspiration. I turned to Charlie and said '***Why don't we treat him with penicillamine***?'. Not surprisingly

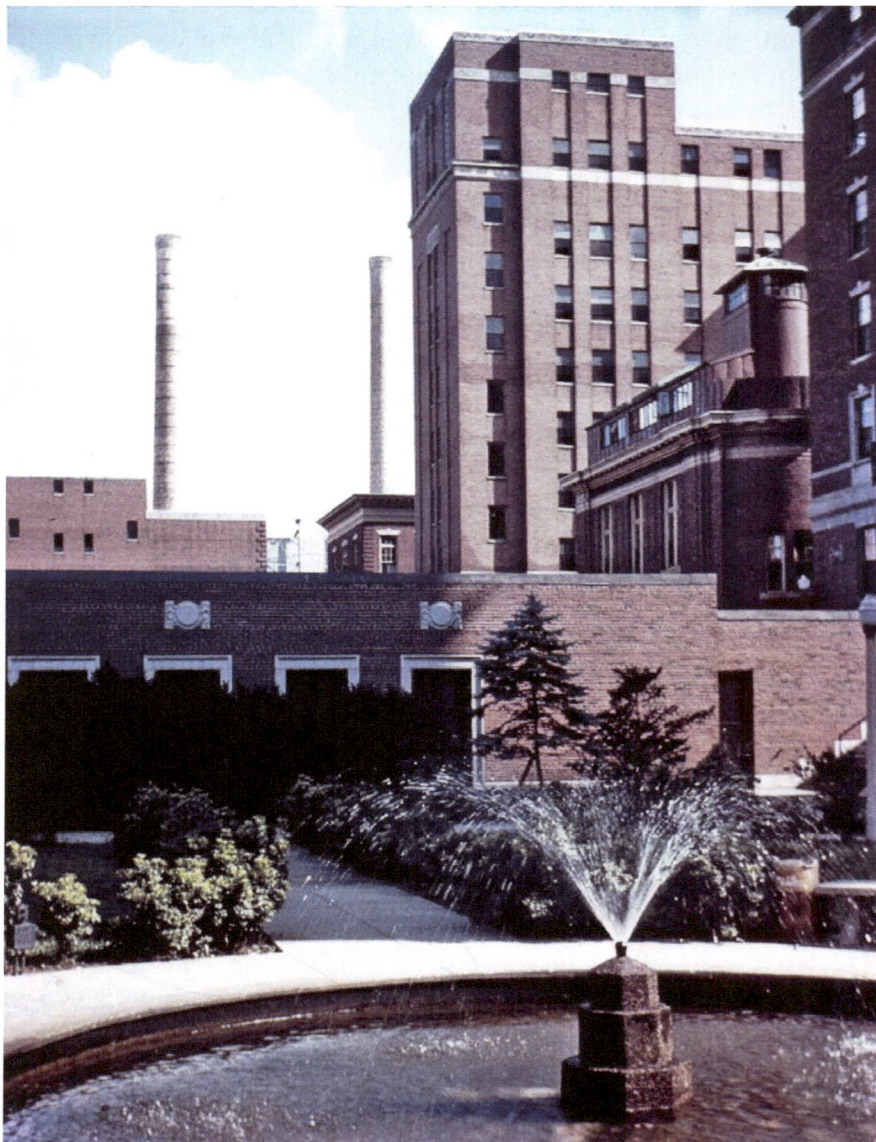

Fig. (2). The 'bridge' at Boston City Hospital in May 1955. The 'bridge was actually the walk way above the corridor joining the Thorndike memorial laboratory, small building left with the neurological wards on the right, not shown in this picture. The Thorndike laboratory was the home of the Liver Unit. It was on this walk way that I had the inspiration that penicillamine might be an effective treatment for Wilson's disease.

Charlie asked 'What on earth is penicillamine?' I explained to him that it was a breakdown product of penicillin, that it could be found in the urine of patients treated with penicillin and that it had the right chemical formula, theoretically, to chelate copper. That is it had a sulphydryl (-SH) group and an amino group (-NH). This combination could form a ring compound with copper. As pencillamine appeared to be readily excreted in the urine this could well be a mechanism for depleting the body stores of the excess metal. In addition penicillamine had the advantage over BAL in that it could be given by mouth; thus it would relieve the patient of the burden of painful injections and might well be more active than BAL. When asked later, by a colleague, where the idea came from all I could do was to point to the sky and say '***Someone up there, perhaps'*** Charlie's immediate response was, 'I think I can get you some. I know Professor Sheehan at the Massachusetts Institute of Technology and he is working on the chemistry of penicillin'. Charlie was as good as his word and a few days later 2 grams of penicillamine arrived on my desk.

Now I was confronted with a new problem, will it be safe to give a dose of this untried compound to a patient.? What was known of its toxicity? The L- form was known to be toxic to rats, the D form appeared to be relatively safe to those animals but it had never been tried on man. If it was safe, how much to give and for how long ? All quite unknown at that time. In those days there were no such things as Ethical Committees from whom to seek permission and approval. I searched the medical literature and found that penicillamine had been given to growing rats with some toxic results; it induced a deficiency of Vitamin B6 (Pyridoxin). However, as already described, penicillamine can exist in two stereoisomers the D-form (produced by the acid hydrolysis of penicillin) and the enantiomorphic L-form. It was the latter which had been used in the rat experiments. I postulated that as the compound found in the urine was the D-form, it ought to be safe. But to give it, untested, to a patient was problematical.. However as it was D-penicillamine that I proposed to give to the patient and as I knew that patients treated with penicillamine all excreted D-penicillamine in the urine it seemed reasonable to assume that it would be safe. I had no intention to use, nor did I have access, to the L-form of the compound. Under these circumstances the ratio of risk to benefit must be taken into account. To give a new untested compound to relieve a headache is clearly unacceptable, to give it to a patient who will die without intervention is another story. I remembered Charles Dent saying to me, '***never give an untried compound to a patient if you are not prepared to take it yourself'***.I decided that, under the circumstances, the correct thing to do was first to take a dose myself and see what happened, but how much? There were no guide lines but knowing that penicillamine appeared in the urine of anyone taking the drug it should be possible to estimate a safe dose. Calculating from the amount likely to be produced in the body from a standard dose of penicillin I estimated that 1 g should constitute a reasonable dose. I therefore divided my precious 2 grams in half; powder is not easy to swallow so I decided to dissolve this in a minimum of water. To my horror, when I added the water, the solution immediately turned a rich blue. Then I remembered a simple chemical fact, -SH compounds give a blue colour reaction with iron salts, bingo, my penicillamine was in the correct reduced form to chelate copper and the colour reaction was due to iron present in the hospital pipes and it had leached into the water. Penicillamine, on standing, can auto-oxidise, that is two molecules of the compound can come together and the two –SH groups combine to form an S-S bridge, thereby removing the ability to bind copper. I therefore plucked up courage and swallowed the somewhat noxious brew, it tasted horrible. The -SH group in penicillamine giving it the same nasty taste as that of bad eggs. The next morning I was alive and well with no undue side effects so it seemed safe to give the remaining gram to Joe. No doubt I discussed what I was doing with him, I certainly never obtained written consent. What I did with impunity in 1955 would certainly not be permissible to day. I doubt very much if any ethical committee would have looked kindly on such an irresponsible research application. Refusal would have set back if not completely aborted my research by many years and also cost many lives. Mercifully the experiment was a success. Joe suffered no ill effects and there was a great increase in the amount of copper excreted in his urine. I reported back to Professor Denny Brown my findings and he, very kindly, found me two more patients on whom to assess the biochemical efficacy of my new drug. These initial studies were simply to determine if penicillamine was able to increase the amount of copper excreted in the urine, they were in no way a test of its clinically efficacy.

The next problem was to find more D-penicillamine. Charlie Davidson again drew on his nexus of connections and approached the medical director of the giant pharmaceutical company Merck, Sharp and Dohme (M.S and D). They did some short term toxicity tests on mice for me and reported no ill effects and they supplied a further few grams of the compound. When I gave a test dose of the new batch to the next two patients I was disappointed to get no increase in copper out put. There, I said to myself, goes a wonderful idea. The result of the first study must have been due to faulty technique. Further thought led to a rush of brains to the head. Perhaps the new batch was auto-oxidised from long standing and no longer contained the –SH group necessary for chelation. By using the simple test of seeking a blue colour reaction with an iron salt I was able to show that, indeed, the MS and D compound had auto-oxidised to tetramethyl cystine and no longer had the free -SH group which gave it its chelating properties. A letter to Merck pointed this out and asked if they could let me have some more penicillamine that had not auto-oxidised. They replied was that I was at fault and the compound was in the active state. I wrote back suggesting they did a simple iron salt test ! This resulted in a further letter from M.S and D. Yes, they admitted that I was quite correct, they were sorry there was none of the active compound available and they hoped *'this will not interfere with your research'*! By this time my year in the US was coming to an end but fortunately Professor Sheehan came to the rescue, he put me in touch with a chemical firm in New York, Mann's Fine Chemicals, who might be able to supply my needs. Indeed they could, they had 50 g of a stable penicillamine acetone compound available. I bought the lot for $50, thereby preventing any one else from pursuing my idea before I could bring it to fruition myself. So, armed with my 50 grams of penicillamine acetonide I set out for home. First stop was Montreal where one of Charles Dent's former postgraduate fellows was now based and with whom I wanted to renew contact. Ironically yet another hurricane was making its way up the eastern shores of the United States and deposited 11 inches of rain on Boston temporarily cutting it off from the outside world, but the floods subsided in time for me to make the journey north. There I joined up with Freddie Flynn and we embarked on the new Cunardar, the Ivernia which had just completed its maiden voyage, and this carried us homeward down the St Lawrence river. I was armed with an idea, a reasonably generous supply of penicillamine and a determination to prove my idea correct.

CHAPTER 2

Progress

With them the seed of Wisdom did I sow,
And with my own hand labour'd it to grow.
The Rubaiyat of Omar Khayyam. Trnas. Edward Fitzgerald.

Abstract: On returning to University College Hospital in London I needed to find patients with this rare disease and supplies of penicillamine to assess its ability to mobilise copper from their abnormal body stores. Three patients were found by my father, Sir Francis Walshe, a distinguished neurologist, and with the small amount of penicillamine available to me I was able to show that in each case penicillamine promoted the excretion of more copper than did BAL. Two patients were returned to their referring physicians but the third stayed with me for over 50 years and made an excellent recovery eventually having three children of her own.

Supplies of penicillamine were secured when I was able to convince the medical director of the Distillers Company, the principal makers of penicillin at the time, to make penicillamine for me.

By the early 1960s reports from my own work and from other centres appeared showing that patients treated with penicillin showed a remarkable improvement in all symptoms.

However Propfessor Denny Brown and Dr Uzman in Boston still believed that Wilson's disease was not due to copper deposition but due to abnormal protein metabolism with abnormal peptides being excreted in the urine. Working with Professor Milne and Dr Asatoor at the Hammersmith Hospital, it was possible to disprove this theory using newer techniques to analyse urine.

In 1957, after failing to get appointed to two different appointments in Oxford I was accepted to a post in the Department of Experimental Medicine in Cambridge.

If the last chapter was the story of the one percent inspiration, the subsequent chapters are the tale of the ninety nine percent perspiration, and much indeed was shed. Having returned to England and to the Medical Unit at University College Hospital, I was confronted with two problems which I needs must solve if I was to pursue this line of research into the treatment of Wilson's disease. One was to find patients with this very rare disease for study; the second, to establish a regular supply of a rare chemical which was not available commercially. My 50 grams of the penicillamine complex would give me a good start but would not last for ever. Having overcome these two problems I then had to show that a drug which could, on a one off basis, increase copper loss in the urine would, if given over a long term, actually lead to a control of the disease or possibly improvement of symptoms with out inducing unwanted side effects. At that time, and it may still be so, the doctrine held by all neurologists was that there was no recovery from a loss of neurones in the brain. If true this would suggest that even if all excess copper was removed only an arrest of progress of the disease could be expected, not a recovery in the control of abnormal movement. However the temporary improvement observed after treatment with BAL suggested that it was reasonable to anticipate that patients could be so helped by the new drug. But before I could initiate this line of research I had to resume my appointment as an assistant on the Medical Unit at University College Hospital and justify my position by work in the wards and out patient clinic. My research would have to be fitted in with the routine by day and using the facilities in Charles Dent's metabolic laboratory first thing in the morning and again in the evenings. The first problem which had to be solved before any progress could be made was to find patients with Wilson's disease on whom my drug could be assessed. Fortunately this proved to be relatively easy for me as my father, Sir Francis Walshe, was Britain's leading neurologist and he persuaded two of his colleagues to allow me to study three of their patients. Two from the National Hospital, Queen Square, both patients of Dr. Dennis Brinton, and one from Dr Michael Ashby at the Archway Hospital in North London. All showed quite advanced movement disorders and had had been treated with courses of BAL without showing significant benefit. When these three patients were tested with penicillamine they all responded with the predicted great increase in copper excretion. Unfortunately Dr Brinton, at the National Hospital, was not sufficiently impressed by these findings and his patients were returned to continue treatment with BAL, I believe one died shortly afterwards from bleeding from veins in the oesophagus, the other was eventually changed to penicillamine, but I never saw her again so I have no means of knowing how she responded to the change. However Shirley, from the Archway Hospital, stayed with me until my final retirement in the year 2000, to become the first patient ever to be put on long term treatment with the new 'wonder drug'. At that time she was a teenager, very severely handicapped with a parkinsonian like disability, bedridden and in need of help in feeding and dressing herself. To be able to treat her I had to prepare from the penicillamine-acetone complex, which I had brought back from the USA, free penicillamine and then pack it into capsules for her to take. This I did in the laboratory, after a busy day in the hospital. In consequence I simply could not encapsulated enough to give Shirely as large a dose as I would have wished. Thus she was treated with only about one third the dose that I would now think suitable for a new patient. However we persevered together and after about nine months she was clearly on the mend. Now, more than 50 years later, she is still taking penicillamine and has brought up a family of three children. There are very few drugs which have to be given continuously over such a long period of time; but without this treatment she would, all most certainly, have been dead within a year.

The next problem was to find a secure a reliable, long term supply of penicillamine. My first thought was to make it myself from penicillin. In the early 1950s penicillin was still relatively rare and expensive drug. However the hospital pharmacy gave me some and I tried to break this down by reacting it with strong acid, as suggested in the literature. All that I succeeded in doing was to produce a sticky mess with the properties of chewing gum and the flavour of bad eggs, no relation to what I needed. After several failed attempts I gave up the unequal struggle and turned to industry. Here again my luck held. At that time penicillin was still made by a fermentation process and the Distillers Company had proved the most successful in this respect. I approached them and their medical adviser, Dr Kennedy, came to see me in Dr. Dent's laboratory on the fourth floor of the Medical School. Dr Kennedy was an asthmatic and the day he came to see me the lift was out of order. By the time he had climbed four flights of stairs he was so breathless that I think I could have sold him almost any hair brained scheme that came into my head. Be that as it may, he was sufficiently impressed by what I had to say and the evidence I provided so that he agreed to try and supply me with penicillamine. Here again I was fortunate and the firms chief chemist, Mr Eaglesfield, was able to work out a simple synthesis and my supplies were henceforth secured. To these two gentlemen I, and many patients, must forever be grateful. When I first showed, in the Boston City Hospital, that penicillamine had real potential as a drug it occurred to me that I should patent the idea but, on second thoughts, I felt that it was more important to publish my findings and make this new treatment available to patients as soon as possible and also to secure my niche in this line of research. Furthermore it is not easy to patent a new use for a known compound; but in view of the fact that penicillamine was later found also to be of use in the treatment of both rheumatoid arthritis and cystinuria a patent might have been worth trying for. As it turned out any enterprising pharmaceutical company who so wished would be able to move into this market with out incurring any of the enormous expenses involved in the production of a new drug. Some, including M.S and D., who had proved less than helpful in the early stages, have subsequently done so, presumably to the benefit of their shareholders. Shortly after my return home I reported my initial findings to a meeting of the Medical Research Society. I doubt if my report set the meting on fire but one distinguished physician was heard to remark that it was a nice bit of serendipity to make such an observation.

The year after returning from Boston I married Ann, a relationship which easily withstood my years absence has lasted us now for over 50 years. We set up home in a very comfortable flat in Hampstead conveniently placed midway between the old Hampstead General Hospital and the Police Station so all our emergency needs would be catered for. We were able to get a first refusal for this most desirable property as Ann was working as a personal assistant in an up market west end house agents. Our first daughter, Susan, was born in St Mary's Hospital the following year.

The medical profession is inherently suspicious, and rightly so, in claiming to cure of a hitherto fatal disease so I needed to show that not only did the new drug cause an increase of copper excretion but that this was from excess body stores of the metal and not merely dietary copper dragged into the body from copper ingested in the diet and then excreted via the urine. I therefore sought the help of Sidney Osborn, the hospital physicist, and asked him if there was a radioactive isotope of copper which could be used to study the movement of this metal in the body. There was, or rather there is, such an isotope known as copper 64 ($_{64}$Cu). Copper 64 emits hard gamma rays and has a short half life of 10.8 hours, that means that half the initial radioactivity has disappeared in that time. Thus it can be followed in the body and urine for approximately 48 hours only, after which time there is so little radioactivity left that it can not be detected. We were the first to show that it was possible to measure the uptake of copper in the liver and its distribution about the body using this isotope. We made a number of model livers of known capacity which would approximate to the size of the liver found in any given patient. These we would fill with a known amount of radioactive copper and by comparing this with the activity found in the patients liver we could calculate the percentage of the administered dose that was taken up in that organ. After we both left University College Hospital we were able to continue our cooperation for many years when I was in Cambridge and Sidney had moved to Kings College Hospital in south London. This isotope, supplied us by the radiochemical centre at Amersham, was of high specific activity, that is only trace amounts of copper had to be administered to get good results. At that time it was very modestly priced and was made available on request, a state of affairs which, unfortunately did not last for ever. After we had both parted from University College Hospital Sidney Osborn collected the radiocopper from the Radiochemical Centre at Amersham on a Monday afternoon and drove up to Cambridge. We prepared it for injection that evening so that we could start our study first thing on a Tuesday morning, this gave us the rest of the week for our investigations. By studying both patients and normal volunteers and also patients with other forms of liver disease we were able to show a significant difference in the handling of copper between these groups. In addition we succeeded in showing that the patients did indeed excrete copper that really was derived from abnormal body store, thus the increased copper we were detecting in the urine really was as a result of depletion of the abnormal body stores of the metal which was causing the disease and did result from treatment with penicillamine.

Later it was possible, using improved techniques, to help unravel some of the problems in understanding the mechanisms of the disease. In addition, thanks to a grant from the Medical Research Council, we were able to get another very much more expensive radioisotope of copper, Copper 67, with a significantly longer half life, approximately 60 hours, which allowed us to follow the movement of the metal in the body, and its rate of excretion, for as long as two weeks. Thus it was possible to demonstrate that normal people started to excrete the injected copper via the bile after about 48 hours whilst the Wilson's disease patients failed to do so. Unfortunately the increased cost and the difficulty in producing Copper 67 meant that it could only be used on very special occasions. Thus most studies had to be carried out with Copper 64. By the early 1960s I found it possible to published a number of articles in the medical literature reporting the marked improvement in patients symptoms as well as improvement in the biochemical tests of liver function brought about by long term treatment with penicillamine. I was also able to report the results of all of the isotope studies up to date. The first of these reports described how Shirley had improved and showing the changes in her handwriting resulted in the Medical Correspondent from the Sunday Times coming to interview me with the assurance that his article, when it appeared, would result in fame and fortune! The article eventually appeared, under the title 'How the wiggles disappeared from Shirley's handwriting' That Sunday morning, shortly after breakfast the telephone rang and a disapproving voice told me, in no uncertain terms, that Dr Kinnier Wilson's name had been incorrectly spelt. And that was the sole result of the article. However the report in The Lancet did convinced a number of physicians about the country that this new approach to managing patients with Wilson's disease was a real advance in treatment.In consequence of this a small but steady stream of new patients were referred to me for confirmation of the diagnosis and for treatment.

Little more than a year after leaving Boston I was back at the City Hospital for a brief return visit. While there I attended the 'Grand Round', where Dr Denny Brown was showing a patient with Wilson's disease. He had been so helpful during my stay the year before that I thought he would have some kind words to say about my work However during that year his deputy, Dr.Uzman, had returned from military service in the US Army and he had other ideas. Indeed Uzman had proposed a new theory about the cause of Wilson's disease; it was due, according to his hypothesis, to an abnormality of peptide metabolism and copper was simply deposited in dead or dying tissues as a secondary effect, it had no significance as a causative agent in the pathogenesis of Wilson's disease. Why he and Denny Brown could not see that this was incompatible with their brief for treatment of the disease with BAL, a drug designed specifically to remove excess copper, as they passionately believed, I could never understand, the logic eluded me. However, armed with Uzman's theories, Denny Brown carried out what must have been a premeditated and well directed demolition of my proposal that penicillamine should be used to treat Wilson's disease. At the time I remembered my father saying that all discoveries go through three stages, first they are not true, then they are not important and finally, we knew that all the time. Mine had already reached the first stage.

Some years later, in 1976, it was possible finally to demolish beyond doubt Uzman's theories in some joint work with Professor Milne and Dr Asatoor of the Westminster Hospital. Using techniques not available to Uzman we showed that there were no abnormal peptides, that the increase in excretion of aminoacids was due to a renal leak and that this returned to normal in well treated patients. Be that as it may, there were, by that time, other centres in the United States working on Wilson's disease which took a more favourable view. In Salt Lake City Dr Cartwright and his team had done important basic work on the role of copper in metabolism and had already mustered a significant number of patients with Wilson's disease on whom they were able to assess the beneficial effect of treatment with penicillamine and as a result he came to realize the possibilities it offered for long term management. A few years later he was quoted, in an article entitled *'Live and let Live'* in no less a journal than The New Yorker, as saying "***The treatment now in use was developed by John Walshe at Cambridge in 1956. His paper 'Penicillamine: a new oral therapy for Wilson's disease is a classic.*'** Actually 1956 was the year of publication of my hypothesis not when the work was done. Another supporter was Dr Scheinberg at the Albert Einstein College of Medicine in New York where he was also making important observations on Wilson's disease and who sadly died early in the year 2009. This initial support he gave me blossomed into a firm friendship which has lasted to this day. In Britain there was less interest in Wilson's disease and Professor Cumings was still the accepted expert and he remained firmly wedded to BAL as the treatment of choice. perhaps not surprisingly as he had been the first to suggest it.

By this time my Professor (Max) Rosenheim decided new blood was needed in the Medical Unit and that it was time for me to move on. First he suggested I apply for a post in the Oxford Medical School, based at the Radcliffe Infirmary. This sounded an attractive proposition, what could be better than an academic job in Oxford, a world class University, a delightful city in an attractive countryside. However, when I looked at the small print of the job advertisement I found that I would be expected to spend my time teaching first year medical students. Not my scene at all, I could think of nothing I would like less. However not to apply would have been a mistake. I therefore did what I was told, an unusual phenomenon, and in due course was summoned to Oxford for interview. On arrival I found I was one of a short list of four candidates. Being, to coin a phrase, 'alphabetically challenged' (the W of Walshe comes well down the alphabet) I was interviewed last. One of the first questions I was asked was 'Do you like teaching?' Should I be honest and say 'No'; which would leave me vulnerable to the next question 'Why have you applied'. To this I could hardly answer 'Well I was told to by my professor' There was a grave risk that such a reply would feed back to him which would leave me in an impossible position. Any other answer might have left me vulnerable to being appointed so, plucking up courage with both hands, I told the truth and said 'No, it was not my first interest'. I felt much safer after this. The rest of the interview went quite well and I was asked no more difficult questions except one about the order of monks in a recently excavated monastic remains in Kent ! When I returned to the waiting room I found myself as one of a company of four expectant candidates, three terrified they would not be appointed and myself terrified that I would. My fears were unfounded, I was told by the chairman that although he committee were much impressed by my credentials they did not think I was the man for the job. I returned, that evening, to London much relieved.

This job failure was followed by another, also at Oxford. Professor Sir Hans Krebs, the very distinguished Professor of Biochemistry, was looking for a clinician to work in his department, having fallen out with the present incumbent. The post was not advertised in any medical journal but was being circulated on 'the old boy's network' and Charles Dent suggested my name. Again I was duly summoned for a further interview. This time it was an informal meeting with Sir Hans alone. We seemed to get on quite well although my interests were not his. I had admitted at the interview that I had not done a biochemistry course as a student, to which he replied to my surprise '*Neither did I'*. Nothing came of this either. Again I was somewhat relieved because my predecessor would still be present and, as I believe, was a powerful figure in Oxford politics, so my own position could have been uncomfortable to say the least. On the drive home to London I was able to observe a total eclipse of the moon. Then a vacancy became available in Professor McCance's Department of Experimental Medicine at Cambridge University as 'Assistant Director of Research' with an honorary consultant appointment at Addenbrooke's Hospital. This sounded a grand title but, what I did not know at the time, assistant directors of research were almost at the very bottom of the pecking order in the University. Such a move, it would seem, was from one ancient seat of learning to another. For this post I applied and, without so much as an interview, was duly appointed. Being of a somewhat cynical turn of mind I could only assume that there were no other applicants for the post. I was very surprised at this appointment in view of my failure to achieve the degree of MD some years earlier and the somewhat acrimonious correspondence with the Regius Professor, Sir Lionel Whitby, that resulted there from; a fore taste of my relationship with the University which were never less than unhappy.

CHAPTER 3

A New Beginning

Every public action which is not customary, either is wrong, or, if it is right is a dangerous precedent. It follows that nothing should ever be done for the first time.
F.M.Cornford; Microcosmographia Academica.

Abstract: Having been appointed Assistant Director of Research to Professor McCance in Cambridge I needed to find somewhere to live and to decide upon a line of research in keeping with the facilities available.. Shortly after taking up this new post I was invited, by the British Council, to undertake a lecture tour in South America. On returning from this I succeeded in establishing the methods I needed to estimate abnormalities of copper metabolism and to recruit patients for my studies. I also continued my work with Sydney Osborn, a medical physicist, and we improved our methods of determining the movement of copper in the body using a short half life radioactive isotope of copper.

Whilst the results of treatment with penicillamine were very encouraging I encountered the problem of a patient developing a severe toxic reaction to the drug. A University biochemist, Dr Hal Dixon, suggested I use triethylenetetramine, a known copper binding compound and this proved safe and effective. For several years we produced this in my laboratory to treat a small number of penicillamine intolerant patients. We also found that an impurity in this compound could induced a disastrous fall in blood pressure. During the course of these studies we moved premises twice, first temporary war time huts in Canhams yard and then the old Low Temperature Research building in the Downing Street site. During this time I also had trouble with the Ministry of Health over the question of prescription charges for my patients.

My first, task before taking up the appointment, was to find somewhere in Cambridge to live. With Ann, my wife, we made several trips up from London in search of a new home. We soon decided we did not want to live in the city; what we wanted was a period house in one of the neighbouring villages. We visited all the house agents and were shown a lot of dross. We did see one house in the beautiful village of Ashwell, probably late medieval, which we hoped to buy but it was under offer and we lost it. We then saw a William and Mary house in the riverside village of Hemingford Grey which had real potential, although it had been sadly neglected for years and needed much doing to it. Ann's former boss, a surveyor, kindly looked at it for us and advised us to go ahead and make an offer. He also undertook to oversee the necessary repairs to the roof and windows. We decided we would do the decorations ourselves, the interior was all municipal green. That was a purchase we have never regretted and it has proved a lovely home in which to bring up our two girls and in which to grow old gracefully together. As the previous owner had died intestate the lawyers held us up for months over settling the final exchange of contracts so we could not move in until the following Easter. The day we moved it was snowing and the builder had still not got all the windows back into the house, it was very cold. We camped in two rooms for several weeks there after whilst the repairs were completed. Originally the house had belonged John Ibbott, who paid off his mortgage in 1703 for the princely sum of £12.11.03 in '*Ye good and lawful monies of England'.* I wish I could have got it at the same price. Our second daughter, Clare, was born in the house two years later.

Thus by the time University term started in October we were still in fact house hunting. We had nowhere to live. One possible solution was to take the temporary accommodation the University offered new appointees. Being a lowly assistant director of research, with little status to boast of in the University, what was on offer was little better than a slum clearance scheme.

This left a somewhat sour taste and my relations with the University never improved over the subsequent thirty years that I remained in their employ. We rejected this housing out of hand. I therefore accepted an offer of a room in the house of the Dominican Friars where I lodged for six months, driving home to London on Friday evenings and returning to Cambridge first thing Monday morning. But it was a good move and allowed us time to find a house we liked, probably dating back to the time of William and Mary. We have enjoyed our home for more than fifty years subsequently. We felt rewarded for our work on essential repairs when, a few years later, it was visited by some members of the Royal Commission on Historical monuments and awarded a star to its grade II listing.

As far as work was concerned my first task was to set up and validate methods for estimating trace amounts of copper in body fluids, also to find the best assay for the copper binding serum protein, caeruloplasmin (Fig. **3**). The significance of this protein had recently been discovered, as already described, by Bearn and, independently, by Scheinberg in New York: Herb Scheinberg was at the Albert Einstein College of medicine and Alick Bearn, an expatriate English physician, was working at the Rockefeller Institute. Herb gave me some help with the assay for caeruloplasmin with a simple kit which we used until I was able to set up a more accurate method, an enzyme assay, recently described in a medical journal, The Lancet. Subsequently it was possible to standardize this procedure with great accuracy thanks to a generous gift of the recrystallised protein from Mme Steinbuch of the National Blood Transfusion Laboratory in Paris: such is the nature of international cooperation in medical research.

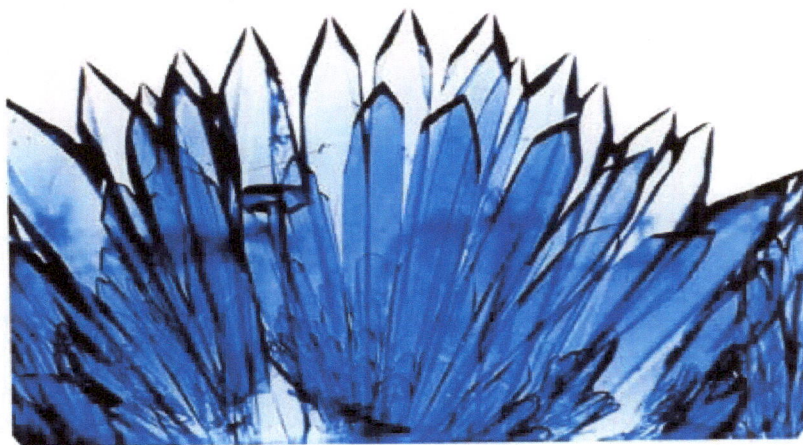

Fig. (3). Crystals of the serum copper-protein, caeruloplasmin. One molecule of this protein carries six atoms of copper. I am grateful to Dr.H. Scheinberg for this picture.

Shortly after arrival in Cambridge I was invited by the British Council to lecture in South America. This caused something of a problem because University regulations did not permit me to be away from my post during term time until I had been in residence for seven years, after which time I could claim sabbatical leave. However thanks to Professor McCance's intervention with the Faculty Board of Medicine an exception was made and I was given leave to take up this offer. In the next two months I visited Argentina, rather a waste of time as there was a general strike including all the doctors, hence I was diverted to Uruguay and then on to my main port of call Chile where my host Hector Orrego could not have been more welcoming. One week end, as his guest at his family's holiday home at Isla Negra on the Pacific coast, I was able to view a total solar eclipse.Later Hector suffered at the hands of the military dictatorship before escaping to Canada where his talents soon allowed him to reestablish himself in medicine. I saw no Wilson disease on that round of visits but confined my activities to my former interest of liver disease.

After my return I had to re-establish my self in Cambridge. Having already validated my laboratory methods it was now possible to study a sufficient numbers of patients, referred from physicians about the country, to publish, in the medical journal The Lancet, evidence that this new treatment with penicillamine for patients suffering from Wilson disease resulted in significant improvement in both their neurological (Fig. **4**) and hepatic symptoms and their biochemical parameters. Time alone would tell if the remission of symptoms, so achieved, would be permanent. About the same time Herb Scheinberg also published similar findings in his larger series of patients. Penicillamine was well and truly launched. There is a somewhat cynical saying that a new drug should be used '*While it still works'*. As subsequent events proved this did not apply to penicillamine, it has continued to work to the present day. Even my severest critics, Professors Denny Brown and Cumings eventually agreed that here was a real advance in the treatment of patients with Wilson's disease. The diagnosis was no longer an automatic death sentence. How long the remission so obtained would last remained to be determined.

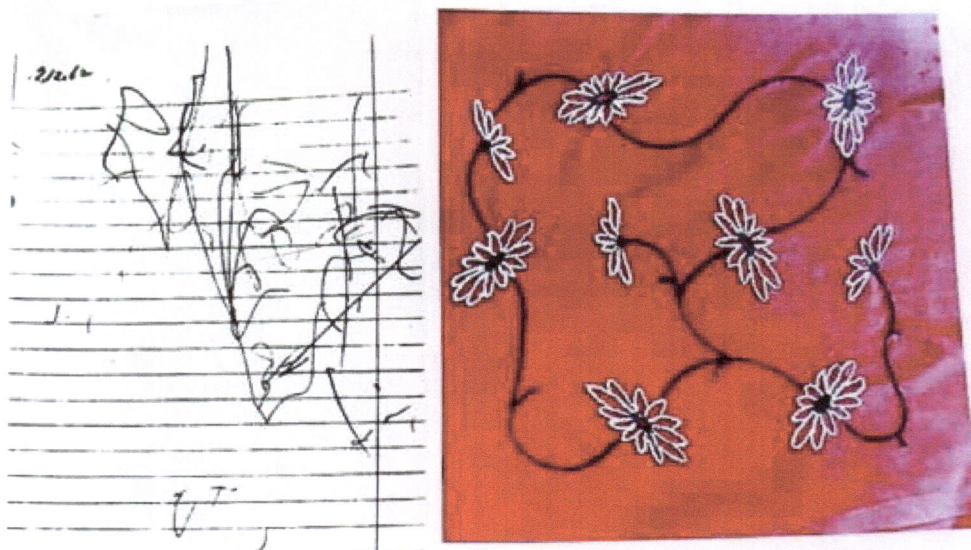

Fig. (4). This shows the attempted handwriting of a teenage Greek girl on a first admission compared with embroidery she completed for me a few years later. This demonstrates the degree of recovery that can be achieved in patients with advanced Wilson's disease.

In 1961 a Dutch neurologist, Dr. G. Schouwink, wrote an MD thesis, of which he sent me a copy, in which he showed that zinc salts could block the absorption of copper from the gut and he suggested that this might be of value in the treatment of Wilson's disease. I must confess that I could not read Dutch but there was an English summary and some excellent diagrams giving the supporting evidence. I had known Dr Schouwink from my previous work on the coma of liver failure and he had also visited me in Cambridge. I wrote back thanking him for the courtesy of sending me a copy of his thesis and added that this should be published in an English speaking journal or else it risked being lost to posterity. I learned later, from him, that having acquired his degree it was necessary to set about earning a living in practice and there was not time for following up this interesting observation. It was however later taken up By Dr. Hoogenraad in Holland and even later by Dr. Brewer in the United States. There was some disagreement between these two as to who had priority in what was essentially Dr. Schouwink's idea ! About the same time my own work suffered a set back when Joy Briggs, my laboratory assistant, left me, her husband had completed his PhD thesis in the University and the couple moved on to pastures new. Joy had been a meticulous worker and kept beautiful notes which remained with me as a lasting legacy. Her replacement, Kay Gibbs stayed with me from that time till my retirement from the University in 1987. Her help proved quite invaluable as events were to prove. She had an excellent background having trained in a hospital laboratory before trying her luck in industry and then at the Agricultural Research Council's station at Babraham near Cambridge. Here she was not happy and was glad to get back to work with a clinical background. Over the years she came to know all of the Wilson's disease patients as well as I did and knew far more about the disease than most physicians Her work for me, as will become apparent, certainly helped save many lives for which she should be given great credit. As the number of young women we treated recovered, got married and had babies a startling fact seemed to be appearing, the first seven successful pregnancies all resulted in the birth of boys: did this mean I had discovered a drug which could be used to control the sex of a child at conception? This would have been a truly explosive discovery. I resisted the temptation to go into print until I had enough figures to be of statistical significance. This, indeed, proved to be a wise decision, future pregnancies showed no such effect, girls were conceived as often as boys. During the 1960s and 1970s one of my chief lines of research continued to be with radioactive copper as this made it possible to follow the movement of the metal in the body after administration either by mouth or by vein. It was also possible to show what happened to it when penicillamine was given. and what effect timing of the dose had on the response. If the drug was given before the copper it promoted the excretion of very much greater amounts than if it was given afterwards.

At first this work was conducted with the help of Sidney Osborn, the hospital physicist now at Kings College Hospital in London. As already described he would drive up to Cambridge, picking up the isotope from the Radiochemical Centre at Amersham, en route. We would then prepare it for injection that evening so as to start work early next day. This particular isotope has a short half life which means it could only be counted in the body for 48 hours, a snag for us but good for the patient as the radioactivity rapidly decayed and left no lasting problems. Initially, whilst we were still based at the old Addenbrooke's Hospital some of this preparatory work had to be done in a broom cupboard under the main staircase ! One early problem occurred when a 14 year old lad from a rather rough background in the North East was admitted. One evening he decamped from the ward into town where he got topped up on cider. Returning to the hospital late and somewhat inebriated he encountered the night sister. The story goes on that he chased her around the hospital with a bread knife. This may well have been exaggerated account of what actually occurred or even apocryphal but there was a distinct atmosphere when I appeared in the ward the next morning.

As time progressed the Department of Experimental Medicine moved from its temporary quarters in the Department of Pathology to some wartime huts, in Canham's Yard (Fig. **5**) just across Tennis Court Road, and slightly nearer the Hospital and where we would no longer be looked upon as guests who had outstayed their welcome. Facilities now became rather better as a new whole body monitor became available in the hospital forecourt so that new techniques could be evolved giving greater accuracy for my radioisotope studies. Later, after a further move to the New Hospital, on the fringes of town, the whole body monitor was no longer at our disposal but I was able to devise an even better technique so as to become independent of Sidney Osborn's help; help for which I will always be grateful. This meant that I had to drive down to Amersham on a Monday to pick up the radiocopper, a pleasant diversion as the journey was largely over back roads and traversing some very pretty country in the Chilterns, one particular woodland had a marvellous carpet of bluebells in the spring.

Later I gave this job to Kay Gibbs. She also appreciated this and it had the additional advantage that she was able to claim a milage allowance for her car when so used. In the actual use of the radiocopper I now received great assistance from Graham Potter and later Karmen Szaz of the Nuclear Medicine Department of Addenbrooke's Hospital.

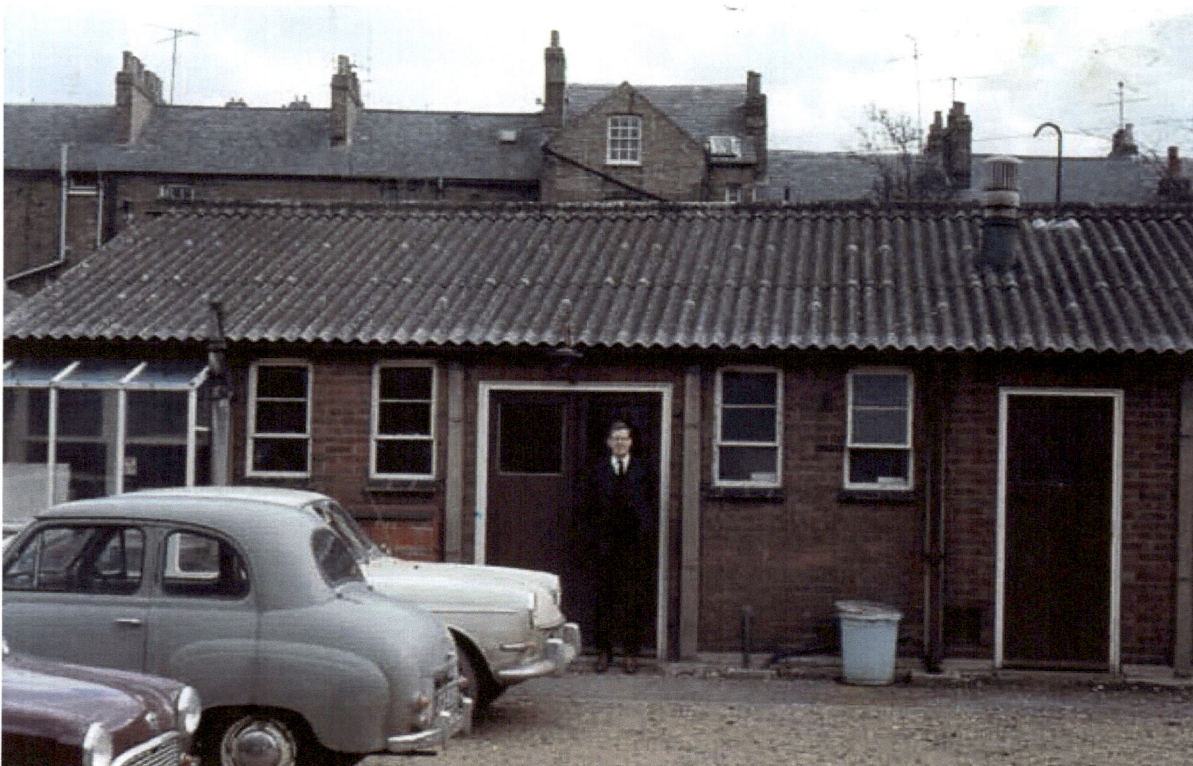

Fig. (5). My laboratory in the temporary wartime huts in Canhams Yard, showing myself in the door. The Department of Experimental Medicine was accommodated here in the mid 1960s before moving into the low temperature research building in the main Downing Street laboratory site.

Events, however, have their own way of shaping research. In the late 1960's progress with penicillamine was severely jolted by the development of an unforeseen drug reaction. Initially I had predicted several possible toxic reactions based on the structural formula of the compound and how this might interfere with normal metabolic processes, damage to the liver or even loss of hair. As none of these had occurred I had been lulled into a sense of false security. The problem which occurred could hardly have been foreseen as it was of an autoimmune nature. In 1969 a lad, let us call him Robert, who had been taking penicillamine for 10 years, presented with a severe kidney lesion precipitated by an immune reaction to the drug. This necessitated stopping treatment for to continue with it would have destroyed his kidneys. I made a number of attempts, trying a variety of strategies, to desensitize him but all failed. I then fell back upon that earlier treatment with BAL. Not surprisingly Robert found this almost intolerable and it as had little effect on his excretion of copper there was no merit in persevering with this approach. Other metal binding agents available at that time were EDTA and a similar compound DPTA, both had to given intravenously which made this an impractical long term treatment. I tried treating him with both of these as a short term measure pending further research. Again neither proved helpful. Thus it was necessary to find a new chelating agent for Robert. If I failed he would certainly die of his Wilson disease or, if I resumed treatment with penicillamine, he would die of renal failure. A conundrum indeed and one which needed rapid solution. With Kay Gibbs help I started to look for an alternative metal binding agent which should be safe to administer by mouth and would promote a great increase in copper excretion in the urine. In a somewhat unscientific way I looked through chemical catalogues seeking compounds which might bind copper, then giving test doses to rats to see what, if any effect, these had. Whilst a number did induce a modest increase in copper excretion none appeared to be sufficiently active to be therapeutically useful.

Then my luck turned. I learned that in the University Department of Biochemistry Dr. Hal Dixon was doing work which might help. Indeed this proved to be true. Hal was a biochemist, not a physician and he knew far more chemistry that I did. He immediately suggested that an industrial chemical used as an epoxy resin hardener might help. The compound, triethylene tetramine, or in brief trien, (later to be marketed as 'trientine') had the exact chemical formula to bind copper. In fact it was known to be a powerful chelating agent for copper (II) ions. Moreover, as Hal pointed out, it was structurally similar to two endogenous polyamines, spermine and spermidine, therefore it was unlikely to be toxic. The only trouble being that trien is an oily liquid, very strongly alkaline and therefore corrosive.

Also the industrial product was only about sixty percent pure, the principal impurity being triaminotriethylamine and this was present in significant amounts. It caused trouble as will be related later. First the crude product had to be neutralised with a strong acid so as to produce a salt which could be crystallized for administration to patients. Hal tried a number of acids, none of which produced crystals and this made purification difficult. The only acid which gave crystalline salt was maleic acid, but maleic acid is in itself an enzyme poison and therefore quite unsuitable. We eventually settled for the salt of hydrochloric acid. Four hydrochloric acid molecules (4HCl) to one of triethylenetetramine gave the best result but I felt that this would overload the patient with chloride and might produce a dangerous acidosis. We there fore settled for 2 hydrochloric acids molecules (2HCl) and this has been the salt used ever since. The parent compound having been thus neutralized was then freeze dried and kept in a desiccator as it otherwise rapidly picked up moisture from the atmosphere and turned in to a sticky brown goo. Armed with this crude, highly impure compound we tested it on rats both for safety and efficacy. To our delight it proved far better at mobilizing copper than anything else assayed so far. Also it gave rise to no untoward effects. Therefore it appeared to be safe to give Robert as a test dose. In practice there was really no alternative. At this time another patient was admitted who had ceased to take his penicillamine as a result of a religious experience and had deteriorated markedly. He also had been subjected to unwise surgery despite my advice to the contrary. As his condition was that of late stage Wilson disease his needs were even greater than those of Robert, he was, therefore, the first to try the new drug. It certainly improved his copper excretion but not his terminal illness. Robert, therefore became the next recipient of trientine, the shortened name for the triethylenetetramine salt of hydrochloric acid. Chemically the response could hardly have been better, the excretion of copper was enormous and there appeared to be no toxic side effects. Thus a new drug was developed for a single patient who had developed a new and unexpected side effect to routine treatment for his rare disease; surely a unique situation. Robert was still taking trinetine 30 years later at the time of my retirement in the year 2000.

Armed with this potential new drug it became necessary to assay its usefulness in as many patients as possible. Thus when patients on routine penicillamine treatment attended for their regular follow up appointments they were each given a single trial dose of trientine and its effect compared with that of penicillamine. To my surprise, in the majority of these, trientine appeared to have relatively much less ability to mobilize copper than did penicillamine. The reason for this I later discovered was that the actual findings depended upon the size of the body store of copper at the time the test was carried out. In untreated patients with a large store of excess copper trientine had a very much greater effect than did penicillamine. After about a year of treatment with either drug the situation was reversed and penicillamine became the more effective. For this and other reasons I postulated that each drug freed copper from a different fluid compartment. The observation had the advantage that the degree of a copper load in any patient could be roughly assessed by comparing the two drugs to see which was the more active. This particular phenomenon seems to have been overlooked by most physicians in choosing the drug of choice for their patients.

There were other developments in the 1960s which require mention. On the clinical side was the realization that Wilson's disease did not necessarily present as a neurological problem of teenagers or young adults as Wilson had believed. It could also occur as a form of liver disease in younger children. This had been pointed out by Dr Uzman in the early 1950s but had actually been first suggested by Dr Bramwell, in Edinburgh, as long ago as 1916. It would be an interesting study to try and trace any possible surviving ancestors of this family to see if they carry, in single dose, a gene for Wilson disease. The children who came to my clinic were most rewarding to look after. I found that if you made friends with them and told them exactly what you needed to do, why it was necessary and how you would do it they always cooperated and thanked you so nicely even after a procedure which must have been, at least worrying to them if not actually painful. I particularly remember one small blonde girl from Yugoslavia who was waiting for a liver biopsy reassuring her frightened mother that all would be well and there was no need to worry! Furthermore I was encouraged by the knowledge that the action I was taking was designed to save the child from a very unpleasant and fatal illness. There is, of course, no certainty in clinical medicine and however well based, theoretically a treatment is, there is always the possibility of side effects and sadly enough, of a few failures.

On the administrative side there was a major change. In 1967 Professor McCance, head of the Department of Experimental Medicine, retired. We had a Festschrift for him which was on the very day that England won the World Cup so all of us from the Department missed that historic television programme ! The unit had been supported by the Medical Research Council and it was the policy of the Council not to renew such appointments but to close down the unit. The University therefore decided the time had come to have a Department of Medicine with its first Professor of Medicine, that is in addition to the long established post of a Regius Professor of Physic dating back to King Henry VIII. I thought that, as an internal candidate with a good research record and an international reputation, I would stand a good chance of being appointed. The University, in its inscrutable wisdom, thought otherwise and I was not even short listed for the post. Though disappointing, this was almost certainly a blessing in disguise. It freed me from administrative work, from the intellectually sterile task of sitting on committees and, eventually teaching medical students basic medicine. It left me free to continue my research unhindered by mundane and essentially, from my personal point of view, non-productive tasks. Also, by now, I had become so specialized that the new head of the department could not reasonably, or in practice, ask me to take on any other duties.

One of the problems that the studies with radiocopper turned up was that the handling of the isotope by the liver varied so much from one patient to another. In some patients the liver sequestered the metal avidly, in others there was scarcely any uptake. Why ? Then, one morning when returning to my laboratory in Tennis Court Road, from the old Addenbrookes hospital the light dawned. I felt like Xenophon when, with the ten thousand, he first glimpsed the Black Sea and cried out, *'Thallatta, Thallatta'*. The explanation was simple, in the earliest, presymptomatic stages of the disease, the liver sequestered copper avidly, as the illness progressed the binding sites for the metal became saturated and copper was distributed elsewhere in the body. Like many good ideas I was left to wonder why this so obvious explanation had not been seen before. Once the liver was saturated with copper the excess metal was deposited in the brain causing the typical destructive lesions leading to loss of control of movements as described in Dr Wilson's original account of the illness.

In the late 1960's we moved again, from the rather primitive temporary wartime huts in Tennis Court Road to new laboratories in the Downing Street Site. Our new quarters were to be, in what had previously been, the low temperature research building. I was lucky enough to get a first class suite with a small office, a main laboratory with an additional room which we used for our radioactive studies. The only drawback was a very tatty linoleum floor, quite unsuitable for isotope work. As the departments isotope officer I was able to condemn this and so get a new floor put down to bring it up to standard for safe working conditions. I also brought over some of the laboratory benches from my old quarters in Canham's Yard and this gave me quite my best laboratory I was ever to occupy. It was the envy of other members of the department (Fig. **6**). Whilst all these changes were going on the number of patients being referred to my clinic continued to increase. In the early 1970s, if my memory serves me aright, I had a visit from two television channels, BBC Overseas and Thames resulting in programmes featuring my work. This led directly to new referrals coming from Europe, first Hungary, then Italy, Yugoslavia Greece.and the Middle East. At the same time physicians in this country who had encountered side effects with penicillamine were referring their patients for treatment with the new compound, trientine as this was not available on the market. This was putting an increasing load on Kay Gibbs who had shouldered the demanding task of preparing and packing into capsules all the trientine needed by our patients. This resulted in a significant slowing down of our other work.

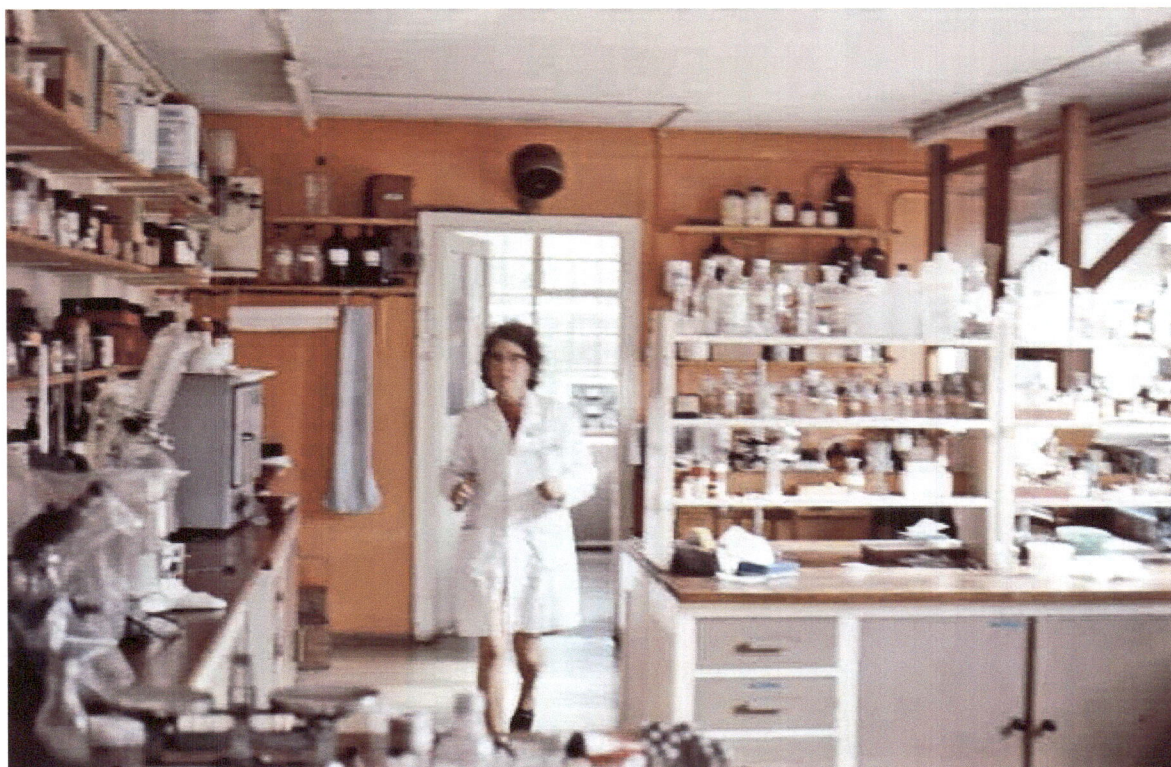

Fig. (6). My laboratory in the low temperature research building. This shows the main laboratory with the isotope room through the door in the background. My invaluable research assistant, Kay Gibbs, in centre picture.

Then, inevitably, we ran into trouble. A young man was admitted from one of the Channel Islands who had become penicillamine intolerant. On arrival he was bedridden and completely helpless. Treatment was immediately started with trientine. As a result of this change of treatment he made a quite remarkable improvement so, within weeks, he was helping about the ward. I was congratulating myself on having achieved one of the most dramatic reversal of symptoms I had ever seen when, rapidly over the course of one long bank holiday weekend, he deteriorated to a state of helpless coma from which, over the course of several months, he never recovered The reason for this I was never able to elucidate. If only CT scanning had been available at the time it might have been possible to throw some light on this state of affairs. All investigations were unhelpful except the finding that his red blood cell count had risen well above the normal level suggesting a possible sludging of the cerebral circulation leading on to brain damage as a rather unlikely explanation. We immediately started to look at the impurities known to be present in the rather crude preparation of treintine which was still in use at that time although the preparation given to the new patient was the same as that taken safely by Robert for several years and to several other patients. My first thought was to do some further studies with rats. As the initial tests had shown no ill effect when the compound was given by mouth I decided to give the crude mixture by injection. To my surprise and dismay the first animal so dosed died very rapidly. I therefore passed on the organs to a colleague in the Department of Pathology, Dr Don Kellaway, who reported that the animal appeared to have died of shock, probably resulting from a catastrophic collapse of the blood pressure. Could my patient also have had a similar episode of very low blood pressure? Considering the chemical nature of what we knew to be the main impurity, triaminotriethylamine, it occurred to me that this compound could act as a ganglion blocking agent which could, in theory, result in such a fall in blood pressure. Studies by Dr Grundy in the Department of Pharmacology proved this hypothesis to be correct. If this untoward toxic effect achieved nothing else, perhaps it would lead to the discovery of a new treatment for high blood pressure? It seemed worth following up this idea. I put the idea to Hal Dixon and we approached a pharmaceutical company with this proposition. This led to discussions about the possibility of taking out a patent. However at about this time there was a real breakthrough in the treatment of high blood pressure and the use of ganglion blocking agents was superseded by newer and better drugs. A potential gold mine bit the dust.What this episode did lead to was a reappraisal of the purity of our drug. Dr Dixon was able to work out a recrystallisation method from absolute alcohol which gave us a very pure product. Absolute alcohol is expensive because of the high duty exacted by the treasury but bought for laboratory purposes the duty is remitted so that this did not lead to a significant increase in our costs and the new method of preparation gave us a much more stable end product. All seemed set fair for future progress. After the recrystallisation the remaining alcohol was no longer one hundred percent pure and of no further use. As customs regulations did not allow us to redistill it the alcohol had to be ditched, which always upset me as it was so obviously wasteful procedure, but was in keeping with yet more bureaucratic regulations. Sometimes the law really is an ass.

One major source of worry, starting in the late 1950s, was the cost of prescription charges for my patients As they were suffering from a disease which, if untreated was invariably fatal, and needing medication for the rest of their lives, these charges presented them with a considerable financial outlay and an extra hardship as many had lost much of their education through the undiagnosed stage of their illness during their teenage years. Saving money by stopping or interrupting treatment was not an option. When charges were first introduced a well meaning, but poorly advised Government advisory body produced a list of diseases exempt from such charges, this list included five hormone deficiency diseases and epilepsy, a quite bizarre list which must have been drawn up by a retired endocrinologist who was already out of date. It seemed to me that the best hope of getting Wilson disease added to the list was to seek the help of my MP, David Renton, MP for Huntingdon. He raised the question in the House, *'Why do patients with Wilson's disease not get free prescriptions?'*. As this occurred during Harold Wilson's premiership it caused some hilarity as other members of the House did not realize this was a serious question about a serious disease. The official answer I received from some lackey in the Ministry of Health was that as there was no cure for this disease there was no point in giving these patients any prescriptions. When I wrote to the Minister pointing out how frighteningly ignorant his advisor was I got no reply. It does not help to point out to a Minister of the Crown that he has been poorly briefed by his Civil Servants. In subsequent years I raised this question with each new administration, each time I got an answer which can be summarised to the effect 'We give free prescriptions to A,B,C,D,; aren't we generous. Hard luck your patients'. My most recent attempt to obtain justice for my patients was to approach Miss Ann Widdicombe, patron of The Wilson's Disease Support Group. The reply she received from Lord Warner (Minister of State (NHS Reform) referred her to a recent report the essence of which was:

'In our response to the report, we have undertaken to review prescription charges and report to Parliament before summer recess next year (2008). The review will look at options to: Revise the list of medical exemptions to prescription charges;
Introduce a flat-rate prescription charge with no exemptions; and
Base exemption to prescription charges solely on income'

I find these a frightening selection of options which look like the forerunner to yet another stealth tax. In Italy free prescriptions are given to all patients with rare diseases, surely we can do as well in this country? Treasury parsimony, on what, in this case would be fiddling amounts of money, can be most depressing. The trouble with health care is that, financially, it is a bottomless pit which was not realized when the Health Service was initiated in 1948. In those days, before high tech medicine, costs were containable. I remember being asked, in the early 1950s, by a very distinguished visiting American Professor of Medicine, Dr Stanley Dorst, what effect State medicine had had on practice and costing. At that time I was able to reply none so far, but as all the money comes from the Government one day they will want to know how it is spent. What foresight ! More recently I wrote to John Major, as MP for Huntingdon, about a Health Service problem in which I stated *'The trouble with the Health Service is that it is run by civil servants who have never seen a sick human being in bed'*. Care of the sick raises a sense of urgency in those at the coal face which it appears to be impossible to transmit to the managers and to the politicians who control the budget. I suspect that the only way such decisions can be reversed is if some public figure takes up the cudgel or some disaster occurs that leads to bad publicity in the press. Most Governments are only interested in votes and a few patients with a rare disease are unlikely to sway the result of a general election. The Government continue to reiterate that they will not tolerate the development of a two tier Health Service. What they do not realize is that they already have one. The best doctors are appointed to the teaching hospitals. Those who fail at this level get appointed to the big town hospitals. The small town hospitals get the rest. This, it seems to me, is inevitable and it is not obvious how it can be remedied.

CHAPTER 4

The Department of Experimental Medicine

Let's all move one place on.
Lewis Caroll, Alice in Wonderland

Abstract: The story resumes with yet another move, the third in all, to new laboratories in the University wing at the New Addenbrooke's Hospital. This had the advantage of being near my ward, the service departments, biochemistry, haematology, radiology and audiovisual aids. It had the disadvantage of removing me from the basic science departments of the University with whom I had had such successful cooperation. In addition my new quarters were much smaller than before and there was no convenient place to see patients. The major problem was the roof. Every time it rained heavily the roof leaked and I had to take unusual action to get this remedied.
However the main problem was the realisation that the impurity in our trientine preparation was not only potentially toxic but, perhaps actually so. This lead to a search for and, eventually thanks again to Hal Dixon, the finding of a solution to the problem. Other activities were a search for a common ancestor to a cluster of Wilson patients centred around the Wash; the search through church records was fascinating but, unfortunately, non productive; the cluster must have been coincidental There was also some work for an ice cream firm who allowed a batch of iced lollies with excess copper onto the market. Finally there was continued work on basic brain chemistry with Sir Rudolph Peters in the University Department of Biochemistry in which we showed how copper might damage the transport of ions through the neuronal membrane.

As I have already described I started work in my new post in the autumn of 1957. I now had my own laboratory and, shortly afterwards, a first class laboratory assistant, Joy Briggs, and with my consultant appointment to the hospital the ability to admit my own patients when and as necessary. I could now peruse my own projects as I wished with out fear of interference. There was one major snag, the University of Cambridge, in its inscrutable wisdom, did not pay its clinical staff at NHS rates, as did all other universities in the country, but at the much lower academic rate, a considerable financial hardship a problem which was later solved by the intervention of the University Grants Committee. At that time the Department of Experimental Medicine was lodged, as a rather unwelcome guest, in the Pathology building in Tennis Court Road. Inevitably it takes a while to re-establish work in new surroundings.

What I did not realize when I was appointed to The Department of Experimental Medicine that was this was, to say the least, a somewhat unusual set up. It was not, in fact a University Department but one which had been established and financed by the Medical Research Council (MRC), in cooperation with the University and with a minority of University staff. The unit had been established specifically for Professor McCance who had done distinguished work on sodium and potassium balances in the body and on nutritional requirements. He had, as his first assistant Miss Elsie Widdowson and these two were very well known and respected for their joint work. Their joint magnum opus was 'The Composition of Food' was indeed a major contribution to knowledge. Elsie, known in the department as 'Mother, was largely in charge of the day to day running of the unit. On the research side there was Dr. Gordon Kennedy, an MRC appointment, usually one or more PhD students, a retired GP in charge of the foetal physiology studies and, of course myself and my assistant representing the University. There was Daphne, seriously disabled, the devoted secretary, Vera, allegedly the dietitian, a department nurse and two ladies in charge of the animal house, the Pledger sisters.

Before the modern era of cost efficiency and Government targets Cambridge was a home for eccentrics. Professor McCance was certainly a distinguished member of this particular

John Walshe (Ed.)

hierarchy. He lived in Bartlow, about 14 miles south east of Cambridge and cycled to and from work every day. When there was a head wind he would choose a route equivalent tacking and was often seen many miles off course. In wet weather he would arrive with oil skins and sou'wester looking, for all the world, like a prewar advertisement for Skipper's sardines. He never used cycle clips to protect his trousers but substituted bits of string which were never removed but kept on all day. During the course of one of my visits to the USA I met a certain doctor, Jerry O'Dell, who I discovered had, in the past, been a postgraduate student in McCance's unit. He told me that these bits of string around the professor's trousers had so irritated him that, on leaving, he presented him with a pair of cycle clips. When I narrated my meeting with Jerry O'Dell, on my return, there was a distinctly frosty silence for several minutes where upon Elsie Widdowson said, in a most lugubrious voice '*Jerry O'Dell, ah yes Jerry O'Dell*' and that was that.

At about 4.30 every afternoon the professor would gird up his loins, go round the department saying, '*Well, I'm off now, anything I can do to help before I go?* As far as I know no one ever took up the offer. On one occasion Ann, my long suffering wife, and her father came to visit me in the department and as they arrived the Professor was just leaving, all geared up for his cycle ride. Ann's father could not be persuaded that this was the professor and not the window cleaner, he was convinced we were pulling his leg. I remember once, when walking down King's Parade seeing McCance standing outside that well known cake shop and eating place, The Copper Kettle. He was staring into the window and, from my angle, reflected in it. It would have made a superb photograph of the hungry tramp gazing at the goodies he could not afford. I did not have a camera with me but I doubt if I would have had the courage to take the picture even if I had. On another occasion, after I had set up my laboratory as a copper free zone for estimating traces of the metal in blood and urine, I needed to set up a method for other studies, requiring copper sulphate as a reagent. To avoid contamination in my own laboratory I decided to set up this method in the large communal laboratory next door to mine and adjoining the Professor's office. This particular method required one of the steps to take exactly ten minutes so I used a pinger to alert me to the exact time for the next step. Towards the end of the afternoon the Professor emerged from his office, just as the pinger went off. '*Ah*', he said, '*So that is what I heard, I thought someone was playing with my bicycle bell*' He always kept his cycle in the laboratory! My own small laboratory had one quite large storage cupboard filled with many of the specimens resulting from the Professor's earlier work. There were many sealed pots with unmentionable specimens but what I thought was of some interest were the packages of high fat toffees. During the war McCance had been an adviser to both the Ministry of Health and to the Admiralty. His advice on the Nation's diet had been remarkably successful, the civilian population may have had to manage on very meager rations but they did remain well nourished and in remarkable good health. His advice to the Admiralty had been on rations for life boats so that torpedoed sailors would stand the best chance of survival. To this end he had formulated the high fat toffee. The ingenious theory being that fat, when oxidized in the body, yields significant amounts of water, thus reducing the needs of this lifesaving essential. I never made trial of the palatability of one of these toffees, twelve years after the war they were most probably well past their 'sell by date'.

Lunch, in the department, was quite a ceremony; we were all expected to attend It was cooked by Vera, the dietitian, and how she produced such excellent meals for such a small charge I shall never know. McCance would sit at the head of the table and take no more than a cup of black coffee; he firmly believed in one gargantuan meal a day which he took in the evening. The lunch would last till two o'clock when the Professor would get up and say '*I must be of, I've got work to do, but you chaps can go on gossiping if you wish*' As soon as he departed we would all heave a sigh of relief scuttle back to work as fast as we could. At Christmas McCance would always give two geese from his farm for the department lunch but to make them go round for the fifteen or so of us was always a task which was never entirely successfully completed. Another story of a Cambridge eccentric which always amused me was of a rather precious Don who was disclaiming to his colleagues in Hall that he never allowed water to pass his lips ! When asked what he did when washing his teeth he simply *replied* '**Well I use a little light Moselle'.** How the falvour of this married up with that of toothpaste history has failed to relate. This is probably beaten by the Oxford story, related to me by Sir Rudolph Peters, of the fellow who suddenly rose from the dinner table in saying '***This can not be Trinity, the food is too good***' and stalked out of Hall.

In 1957 Adenbrooke's Hospital was still a small town hospital with a limited staff. Although Professor McCance was entitled to the use of seven beds in the hospital he very seldom used them so they were readily available to me. He had a distinctly brusque way in discussing cases with his colleagues which did not make for popularity. On one occasion I overheard a telephone conversation in which he said '***You chaps only call me into help when you have made a mess of it***' Thus being a member of this team made the rest of the hospital staff suspicious of the Professor's associates. What he had to say may well have been true but this was not the way to make friends and influence people. My own approach, when referred a patient who had been inexpertly handled, was always to say this was a difficult problem but by doing such and such investigations I think I have sorted it out. Such a reply would not offend the referring doctor and gave a much better chance of him sending further patients to my clinic.

On the purely nonclinical research side there was Gordon Kennedy, I forget what his particular interest was, but it did not impinge on mine. I think he looked on me as a possible dangerous rival to head the department after the Professor retired, but this was never an option as it always was MRC policy to close down such small units when the founder retired, other workers being relocated. This did not worry me as I had a University appointment and after completing my six year appointment as an assistant director of research I was appointed Reader in Metabolic Disease which gave me life tenure. McCance's interest had turned from electrolyte balances and dietary requirements to foetal physiology, for which the retired GP was employed. The studies were carried out on piglets raised in the Professor's own farm and for this purpose a van had been converted into a mobile laboratory so it could rush to the scene when a sow was about to farrow. I could never quite understand how a retired GP, with no research training, working in a makeshift laboratory, which could only be described as Heath Robinson in construction, could possibly hope to make important and valid advances in this difficult branch of science. As far as I know nothing of scientific importance ever came from this line of work.

After McCance retired the University established a professorship of Medicine and appointed Ivor Mills from London. I had applied for the post but did not even reach the short list. I think Ivor found Cambridge difficult compared with working in a London teaching hospital, after all the University had been going for 600 years and this resulted in a good deal of inertia which he could not grasp. For the first few years he would occasionally 'cry on my shoulder' over the difficulties he had with the faculty Board. He carried round with him a list of all the Professorships of Medicine in the country with the retiring dates of the present incumbents in the hope of moving on, but this never came off. From my point of view his appointment meant no change, I went my own sweet way, but life, with out McCance, was distinctly duller.

It must have been after this new dispensation that I started a research project into the basic biochemical defects induced by copper with that very distinguished biochemist Sir Rudolph Peters. My first association with him had occurred some years earlier, in fact shortly after I had returned from my year in Boston. I was still worried about the theoretical, basis of my work on the chelation properties of penicillamine. I had decided to go to the *fons et origo* of metal binding in medicine, it was Sir Rudolph who had led the Oxford team that discovered BAL at the beginning of the war. At that time he had retired from his post in Oxford and was working at he Agricultural Research Council's laboratories at Babraham, a few miles south of Cambridge. He agreed to see me and I drove up from London to spend a very useful afternoon with him. He gave advice freely and was most supportive of my work. By coincidence one of my colleagues from The Thorndike laboratory, a keen American researcher, Dr Norbert Frankel was spending a sabbatical year with Sir Rudolph, a year he greatly appreciated and enjoyed to such an extent that he determined to return to Cambridge when his next sabbatical was due in seven years time. By another strange coincidence it was when I renewed by connection with Sir Rudolph that Norbert had returned to Cambridge for what turned out to be a disastrous year, he suffered terrible health problems and had to return early to the States.

By this time Sir Rudolph had moved on from Babraham and had a laboratory in the University Department of Biochemistry in the Downing Street site, conveniently near the Department of Experimental Medicine, where he was doing important work on lethal synthesis. On this occasion I approached him once more to seek his help in confirming a theory that copper was blocking an enzyme in the cell wall which controlled the movement of metals into or out of the cell. He readily agreed to help and I would visit his laboratory in the Department of Biochemistry and we would measure enzyme activity in very thin brain slices. As a result of these experiments we were able to show that one of the key enzymes, controlling the movement of sodium and potassium into and out of cells was indeed blocked by copper and we were further able to show that direct injection of copper into the brain induced convulsions. Attempts to neturalise this toxic action of copper demonstrated that, under these conditions BAL was more active than penicillamine though this did not necessarily mean that such was the case in man. So keen was Sir Rudolph on these experiments that, on occasions when he had to leave early for one of his many commitments in London, that he would ring me up to find how the work had proceeded after he had left. During the course of one experiment he said to me that he thought that clinical research was a most difficult discipline because it was almost impossible to control the variables; shades of Charles Dent's advice about the importance of having only a single variable in any experiment. However with care and simplification of the experimental protocol it is often possible to achieve this. For instance does a given dose of penicillamine increase urine copper excretion or not; one question, one answer.

One interesting side line that came up was when we were asked to find out if oysters from the estuary of a Cornish river contaminated with copper could be treated to make them edible. As they came out of that particular estuary they had picked up so much copper that they were small and green with a nasty taste, quite unfit for the table. To make them marketable they had to be collected and transferred to another river and left for many months to clean themselves up. The question we were asked was could this process be speeded up by adding a chelating agent to the water in which they were submerged. We rapidly showed that oysters did not like BAL at all and that penicillamine only removed copper so slowly that it was not a viable commercial proposition to use this technique, in fact we were not able to help on this problem. My work with Sir Rudolph did not alter the approach to treatment of patient's with Wilson's disease but did throw some further light on the pathogenesis of the illness and to that extent it was well worthwhile. This type of cooperation with another University Department would become much more difficult after we moved to the New Addenbrooke's Hospital on the fringes of town. If one drove back into town there was no where to park a car and public transport was too slow and infrequent to be of use.

This threatened move, in fact, took place in 1974, the third in all, to the new Addenbrooke's Hospital on the southern fringes of the town. This had both advantages and disadvantages. The gain was that my laboratory was near the wards, the hospital routine laboratory and other service departments. The disadvantage was that the space available was much reduced. There was no office and no place to see patients, furthermore we were now divorced from the main University laboratories making cooperation with these much more difficult. At the same time the University bit the bullet and established a clinical medical school as opposed to the previous rather nebulous postgraduate school. This brought one huge benefit, the University Grants Committee (UGC), before funding the new clinical school, stipulated that clinical staff should receive full rates of pay. I was able to replace my car !

The new Medical School was based in a University wing embedded in the new hospital. This had certain idiosyncarsies, as became apparent with the passage of time. For instance when one of the light bulbs in my laboratory failed the correct procedure was for me to apply to the department administrator for a new bulb. He would then apply to the head electrician of the hospital. After hospital working hours were complete, that is in over time, two electricians would come to my laboratory, one with a ladder and one with a basket full of electric light bulbs. The one with the ladder would solemnly hold it, to comply with health and safety laws, whilst the other climbed to the dizzy height of three or four steps. He would then change all 8 bulbs in the ceiling as this was more cost effect simply than changing the dud one. The logic of this eluded me as did certain of the activities of the University. After this happened a couple of times I decided to go to Wolworth's and buy some bulbs and change them myself. This meant that the work was done by non union labour. Had the electricians known of this they would almost certainly have gone on strike. The hospital unions were very militant at the time and at one time even tried to control admissions. Eventually the problem was solved by changing all the light fittings to fluorescent strips. A further major problem arose because the medical school was set on the top floor of the wing. My laboratory had a ceiling of perforated metal squares. After several years, when it rained heavily, water would come through the perforations like a shower bath. This meant I had to cover my books and sensitive equipment with plastic sheets. Complaints about this fell upon deaf years. Finally I decided to take more aggressive action. I set up a collecting system and one very wet day collected water at the rate of a litre an hour. I then informed The Cambridge Daily News who wrote an article on this pointing out, on my suggestion, that as all the electric wiring ran between my ceiling and the roof so that any defect in the insulation could result in a short circuit and the whole building going up in flames. This spurred the University to action. At great expense the roof was treated to make it weather proof. When the work was completed the workmen swept the remaining debris away, thus blocking the gutters and some of the down pipes. Next time it rained heavily the Professor's office flooded doing significant damage. I must confess sympathy was not the first sentiment that came to mind.

Having established my self in my new quarters it was possible to resume work on both the care of patients, research into the mechanism of their disease and the best possible management. At this point, in the spring of 1975, when we had 7 patients on our new drug all of whom had to be supplied by the efforts of Kay Gibbs, a further difficulty arose. The crude source material of triethylenetetramine had previously been purchased from one of two sources, Hopkins andWilliams or British Drug Houses and, as we subsequently found out, both had bought this in from the American company, Union Carbide. We had to locate a new supplier. We found this in Ciba-Geigy, conveniently placed in near by Duxford. We later discovered that their material was bought in from the American company Dow Chemicals. Our purification procedure remained the same although the final yield of crystals from the new material was slightly less than previously. We therefore proceeded to supply our 7 patients by post as here to fore. Then two new patients were admitted both of whom had developed bone marrow problems on penicillamine; Eve from the North of England, Nicholas from the Norfolk marshland. To my dismay both Eve and Nicholas, shortly after starting treatment, developed acute, severe renal failure. As far as we could surmise this had to be due to a minute trace of a toxic impurity not removed by crystalisation. All patients were immediately written to and advised to stop taking their treatment pending a reappraisal of our purification methods. Six of these patients had been on treatment for a sufficiently long time to be satisfactorily copper depleted so that they could safely be left without their drug for weeks, or perhaps even months. But one of those on the postal list and our two new patients were in urgent need of medication. I called in the help of the University Department of Chemistry but, even with their sophisticated analytical techniques, they were unable to answer the question, what was the new toxin? It must have been very damaging to kidney function in minute amounts. Why the other 7 patients who had received postal supplies were not similarly affected remains a mystery. We shall never know what this toxic effect was due to. Next, Nicholas developed another complication of his Wilson disease and had a massive and fatal bleed from varicose veins in his oesophagus. As a result of this tragedy it was possible to obtain a small amount of kidney tissue for microscopic examination and this demonstrated the location of the lesion which, as we has suspected, was in that region of the kidney controlling the amounts of water and salts to be excreted.

These events led to a desperate search for yet another manufacturer of 'triethylenetetramine', eventually this proved to be Aldrich Chemicals. Their material was put through our purification process and tested on rats with out any ill effect. I then had to make a difficult decision would it safe to give this to Eve who was, by now, desperately ill. If I did nothing Eve would certainly die of untreated Wilson's disease and not in the distant future: but was it ethically acceptable to treat her with a compound which might still contain trace amounts of an unknown toxin? I decided that the latter course would be the lesser of two evils and which offered the only hope of a cure. By this time Eve's kidneys had largely recovered from the earlier insult. Treatment was cautiously reintroduced and her kidney function monitored daily and in detail. To my immense relief the drug was well tolerated and there were no ill effects. Supplies could be resumed to all those patients on the postal list as well. At the same time Eve's response could be watched with both hope and reasonable expectation. Some weeks later she had made an excellent recovery and I was able to discuss with her the prospects of returning home. To my surprise she requested a gynaecological consultation. This being quite outside my field of expertise I made the necessary arrangements. The report from the gynaecologist was, to say the least, surprising indeed. Eve was 8 weeks pregnant. The date of conception could be safely dated back to a visit from her husband some weeks earlier. It is amazing what can go on behind the curtains in a busy ward. Exciting though this finding might seem as it first appeared it raised yet further unexpected problems. Eve was being treated, apparently successfully, with a copper depleting regime. It had been well known to the veterinary profession for many years that lambs born to sheep on a copper poor pasture developed a disease known as sway back, that is a condition in which nerves are not properly formed and the animals do not have control of movement. Would Eve's baby be similarly affected? This did not appear to be a great risk, other Wilson's disease patients treated with penicillamine to remove copper and had babies which were normal so this was not a particular source of worry. However this was a new chemical she was receiving with other unknown possible side effects on the foetus. There was no evidence to suggest whether or not it was teratogenic. Moreover the drug was being given at the most dangerous time in foetal development, the first few weeks of pregnancy. Indeed it was at this stage in foetal development that thalidomide had caused so much damage to the unborn child. Again I was able to call in help, the great advantage of working in a University Department of medicine. Miss Hilda Bruce was expert in this field and she carried out studies on pregnant mice which appeared to show that the drug might be safe, always remembering that thalidomide only showed its potential for harm when tested on several different species. At that time ultrasound scanning during pregnancy, to demonstrate the state of the foetus, was not available so that I had no alternative but to await the remaining seven months to find out if all was well. Happily it was, Eve had a normal healthy boy. Testing of his cord blood reassured me that, although he was, by definition, a carrier of the Wilson disease gene, he did not have two abnormal genes and was therefore not going to develop the same disease as his mother.

Another development in the 1970's was the arrival of the first of the CT scanners. This enabled me to look at the brains of my patients to assess the amount of damage done by the accumulation of copper. In his original description Wilson had shown that areas of cell death had led to the development of cavities in those areas of the brain controlling movement, the so called basal ganglia. His pictures also showed, though he did not comment on it, that the cerebral cortex, that is the outer layers of the brain, were also atrophic. It has long been neurological dogma that there is no recovery in the central nervous system so some of the findings made by this new technique came as something of a surprise. By cooperating with Dr Williams in the radiology department of Addenbrooke's Hospital we studied all patients coming to my clinic on their first attendance and on regular follow up visits. As a result we were able to publish the first study of the brain in Wilson disease using this new scanning technique. The first pictures obtained by this technique, compared to later models, were rather crude. Never the less we were able to show that the lesions visualized in these pictures demonstrated what Wilson had led us to expect, damage to the basal ganglia. However what was remarkable was that, as the patients improved, the cavities in the motor centres disappeared; a quite unexpected observation and one since confirmed from many other centres using both the CAT scanner and more recently by the use of the even more sophisticated MRI scanners.

The year 1977 proved something of a high point. I was awarded the gold medal in therapeutics of the Worshipful Company of Apothecaries, an ancient City Livery Company dating back to the reign of James I. On the day of the award I traveled with Ann, my wife, to London, there we were met by Dr Hugh Lyle who, in a previous post as Medical Director of Dista Products, had been a firm supporter of the development of penicillamine; he had also made possible the Trinity Hall conference to celebrate 21 years of the drug, to which I will refer again later. After a refreshing tea at Brown's Hotel we set out to get a taxi to the Apothecaries Hall for a 6.30 start. Unfortunately, at that time of day taxis were at a premium, and there was some delay before we caught one. Almost unbelievably the Taxi driver had no idea where, in the city, the Hall was to be found, and he added somewhat surprisingly '*These city companies are always changing their addresses* !' When we thought we must be reasonably near the Apothecaries Hall we eventually decided to abandon him and walk. To my chagrin we were met by a posse from the Apothecaries sent out to look for us as we were late. On entering the Hall the meeting had started in my absence and the peroration in my honour was already being delivered. A more embarrassing situation it would be hard to imagine. Every board creaked as I walked to the front of the hall with every disapproving eye fixed on me. It was one of those occasions when one wished the ground would open under one's feet. I discovered afterwards that we had been misinformed and the meeting was in fact called for 6 o'clock, but that hardly helped. I wrote a groveling apology to the Master and felt some kind of rejoinder was called for, but it was not forthcoming.

About this time I was side tracked on a fascinating, but ultimately disappointing line of research. I have already mentioned Nicholas whose home was in a Norfolk village near the Wash. By chance, at about the same time, two more patients were referred from this region, each from a village within four miles of the original one. The sort of distance a village lad could walk on a summer evening to meet his girl friend and, as a result of a tumble in the hay, spread his genes. Was there a common ancestor ? It did not seem an unlikely state of affairs and one which I decided to follow up. So, during several summers, Kay Gibbs and I would take off, if and when routine work permitted the time, to the marshland villages and trail through the church records of births and marriages to seek this elusive progenitor of this particular disease cluster. I had the impression that some of the vicars of these churches were a bit tired of individuals trying to trace their ancestors, but when I explained the nature of my quest, they could not have been more helpful. Some, in fact, were too helpful as they would trail through the records with me not knowing exactly what I was looking for. The further back we took the quest the further apart the ancestors spread. It was impossible to find a link but this did make a pleasant diversion from routine, it also gave me an excuse to visit the splendid marshland churches of the district. We visited many families, built up some large family trees and took many blood samples to look for carriers of the gene. The available technique, at that time, was not very specific but better than nothing. We also involved the help of Dr Ruth Sanger, sister of the Nobel laureate who we hoped, as a blood group expert, might be able to help in tracing the gene. We hoped that it might be possible to link the Wilson disease gene with one of the blood group genes thus imparting greater accuracy to ancestor tracing and, hopefully, helping in the search for the Wilson disease gene. We found that in one family under study was, by coincidence, also known to Dr Sanger as one member was the carrier of a very rare blood group gene of great interest to her.

In another family we managed to trace a member who gave us a fascinating insight to a now forgotten aspect of local history; the hiring fairs. I had never heard of these. Apparently up to the time of the first world war a farm labourer would attend spring fares in the local market town and wait to be hired by a prosperous farmer to work his fields for the year. He would then load his family and his possessions on a cart, move to the his new employer and live in a tied cottage for the year. The next year the procedure would be repeated and he might well move to another farm in a different part of the county. Uncle George, as we came to know this family member, told us how he had moved as far afield as Chatteris in Cambridgeshire, some 30 miles away,! and it was easy to see how a gene could be spread quite widely by this method. Two points did come up, one was the finding of three sisters who, in the 1880's migrated to Australia and later gave rise to a family suffering from whispering dysphonia. In another family we found a Suckling in the ancestry. The Sucklings are a family with a long history in Norfolk as instanced by the medieval Suckling Hall in Norwich and the fact that Nelson's mother was a Suckling from Burnham Thorpe, near Kings Lynn and in the very centre of my particular area of interest. Could I trace the Wilson disease gene back to Admiral Lord Nelson. I could then have described him as one eye, one arm and one gene. It was a fascinating thought, but not medicine. This line or research was going nowhere and, before 1800 the church records were becoming increasingly difficult for a non-expert to read. Reluctantly I decided the time had come to quit.

The 1950's and 1960s might well be described as the boom time for patients with Wilson disease. The successful research initiated in the early 1950s led to an increased awareness of the illness and to greatly increased diagnostic accuracy. The condition was clearly not as rare as had been previously thought, the accepted calculated incidence had fallen from one in a million to one in thirty thousand of the population. As time moved on referrals to my clinic were reaching the maximum I could cope with, particularly as Kay Gibbs was spending more and more time simply making and encapsulating trientine. Fortunately some relief was at hand, the hospital pharmacy agreed to take over the task using the purification method Hal Dixon had perfected and which we had proved to be satisfactory at a practical level.This was a courageous action on the part of the principal pharmacist. The drug was unlicensed, had not been approved by any ethical committee nor had the hospital administration been consulted. Such a state of affairs could not remotely be envisioned today. Who, in addition to myself, would have been held responsible for any unforeseen disaster; would this have involved the pharmacist ? I have no idea but I suspect it might well done so. However I can easily conceive how some learned judge, quite unaware of the difficulties involved or of the human situation, would have uttered words of condemnation to a hushed and expectant courtroom, which bore no relationship to the reality of the problems as they existed in the real world.

As I have said before, from time to time diversions, not directly related to the main line of research, cropped up. One such, unlikely as it may sound, involved a major ice cream manufacturer. One morning I had a phone call from their legal adviser, would I defend them against a claim for negligence. Being cautious I said I would give them the benefit of my expertise if they would give details of the basis of the claim. The story was that a young mother had bought her toddler an iced lolly which had made the child violently sick. Being a perspicacious lady she immediately took the remains of the lolly to a public analyst who reported high levels of copper. I forget the exact figure but it certainly sounded to me to be toxic. Mother thought this wrong and demanded compensation. My immediate reaction was that she had a good case so my reply was that I would look into the literature of acute copper poisoning and report back. Copper is certainly a toxic metal and in the form of copper sulphate it is said to be the commonest method of suicide in India. That distinguished biochemist, Sir Rudolph Peters, once told me that one part in a million was sufficient to kill a gold fish which left me wondering how any of these creatures had survived. I easily found a number of reports of water from corroded copper heaters causing severe gastric upsets. My next move was to go and buy some iced lollies and analyse them for their copper content. In all this proved to be very low and bore no relationship to that found in the toxic lolly. Further enquiries unraveled the problem. Iced lollies are made in copper moulds. The mixture for the lollies contains a relatively high concentration of citric acid as part of the flavouring. Citric acid can attack and bind the copper in the molds but, under normal conditions contact between the lolly and the mold is too brief for the reaction to go ahead, but in this particular case a batch had been left standing over the week end leading to the very high copper level in the lolly in question. The case was clearly indefensible and so I advised the ice cream company. What I was left wondering was what happened to the rest of the batch? Why were there no other similar cases reported ? Perhaps the other victims were not sufficiently street wise or did not put two and two together and realize the cause of the vomiting.

CHAPTER 5

Progress Despite Bureaucracy

Say not the struggle naught availeth
The labour and the wounds are vain,
The enemy faints no, nor faileth,
And as things have been they remain.
Arthur Hugh Clough

Abstract: Although the hospital pharmacy had taken over the production of trientine this drug needed to be put on an official basis with production by a pharmaceutical company. None, however, were interested. A letter to the British Medical Journal aroused some interest but no positive result. In 1976 I convened a conference in Cambridge to which all interested groups were invited to discuss this problem. An unexpected result was that the Department of Health agreed to take out a product license and that the Government Chemist would test the final product for purity if a manufacturer could be found. A small chemical firm Cambrian Chemicals undertook the manufacturer and Rupert Purchase, their principal chemist worked out a large scale method for production. However It took several more years of correspondence with the Department of Health to overcome the bureaucratic baffles and to obtain the necessary product license. This was achieved successfully in 1985, shortly before a similar license was issued in the United States.

Basic work had continued during this time. This included studies with radiolabelled penicillamine to determine its rate of absorption from the gut, distribution in the body and rate of excretion in the urine. Later similar studies were conducted with radiolabellesd trientine. One problem remained, and still remains unsolved. Why does a small percentage of patients fail to respond to any of the currently available lines of treatment. Can it be due to a particularly unfavourable gene mutation?

By the late 1960s an increasing number of toxic reactions were being attributed to penicillamine and this was causing anxiety amongst those physicians using it. In addition to Wilson's disease penicillamine had also been found, for different reasons, to be of value for patients with cystinuria and rheumatoid arthritis and was being tried in a wide variety of other diseases. This called for a meeting, held at the Royal Society of Medicine in 1968, in which all aspects of toxicity were discussed. This in no way decried the valuable contribution it had made to therapy. Indeed the chairman, Professor M.D. Milne, Professor of Medicine at the Postgraduate Medical School at Hammersmith Hospital, said, in his closing remarks '*I would like also to add my voice of thanks to Dr Walshe in appreciation of his early work with this very remarkable drug. It is not, in my experience, very often that formulae of drugs give almost predictable therapeutic responses and I think that this was a very great achievement in relation to penicillamine*'.

At a later meeting convened to up date work on the potential of penicillamine, held at the same venu, the new chairman, Dr. I.A. Jaffe from the New York Medical College, said, in his opening address, *It is now nearly 20 years since Dr. John Walshe discovered penicillamine and introduced it into the treatment of Wilson's disease. He could hardly have appreciated at that time that he had opened a pharmacological treasure chest, the contents of which a re not yet fully realized.*'

By the middle of the 1970's it was becoming apparent that trientine had an important future as an alternative treatment for patients with Wilson disease particularly for those patients who had become penicillamine intolerant. The logistics of preparing an unlicensed drug and sending it out, all over the country and to the occasional overseas patient, was becoming insupportable.

A solution had to be found. In 1975 I wrote an impassioned letter to The British Medical Journal (BMJ) detailing the problem. I quote here extensively.

Sir, It is almost twenty years since I first started to investigate the possibility of using penicillamine in the management of Wilson's disease, I do not wish to launch into a detailed account of the various and not inconsiderable obstacles which had to be overcome before this new drug was accepted into the pharmacopoeia.....That it has proved a major breakthrough in the management of Wilson's disease can hardly be denied and it is of interest that this drug has been found to be of value in other heavy-metal intoxications and a number of other unrelated diseases – namely cystinuria, rheumatoid arthritis, certain diseases of collagen, and perhaps macroglobulinaemia. It would seem highly improbable that, under present day conditions, such a puny infant would have blossomed into such a robust member of the therapeutic community...Penicillamine, like all other active drugs, has certain undesirable side reactions To some extent it has proved to be a veritable Pandora's box and in a recent leading article you listed the widespread and varied toxic reactions which must be set against penicillamine... For those patients whose disease can be managed by alternative methods this is no great disaster, but for patients with Wilson's disease withdrawal of treatment is tantamount to a death sentence. In 1966 I was confronted with this very problem when a youth of fifteen years, who had been taking penicillamine for Wilson's disease for six years developed the nephrotic syndrome. Two attempts at desensitization proved unsuccessful but eventually the situation was saved by the introduction of a new orally active chelating agent triethylenetetramine dihydrochloride. Subsequently it has been necessary to transfer three more patients to this form of treatment... Treatment of these patients, over the years, has been continued simply because the purified drug has been prepared in my laboratory... No pharmaceutical company has seen fit to undertake its production. This is hardly surprising in view of the thalidomide disaster and its unfortunate repercussions, and because of the enormous expense of testing and clearing a new drug through the Medicines Commission... For a private individual to prepare and supply a drug for clinical use must be legally hazardous whatever the indications may be. Fortunately the situation has not yet been tested in the courts but to quote a statement I have made elsewhere, 'The mind boggles at the thought of what a learned judge might say should the experiment prove a failure.'... It might be argued that it is the duty of the Minister in charge of the Health Service, as laid down by Parliament, that such treatment, if it does not put an unreasonable load on the country's resources, be made available to those patients requiring it. Meanwhile the question arises as to what will happen to these patients should I retire from the scene or should a product license not be issued. Are they to be allowed to die of a readily treatable disease because no one is prepared to supply, or worse still is permitted to produce, the necessary medication. Such a refusal would be little better than an act of legislative homicide. I shall appreciate enlightenment in this dilemma'.

What I did not know at the time, but to which my attention has recently been drawn by Rupert Purchase, was that Dr Donald Gould, a medically trained science writer saw this letter and publicized it in The New Scientist in September of the same year. The solution he suggested that might solve this problem was the implementation of a Labour Paarty committee recommendation that, '*The state should acquire an existing pharmaceutical company to compete with private industry. A state owned firm might be charged with the duty of producing essential but unprofitable drugs. And in such very special cases the rigorous requirements of the Medicines Act could sensibly be waved*' Cloud cuckoo land ? As this reached much wider audience than my letter in the British medical Journal it was almost certainly his letter, not mine that led to a number of enquiries from pharmaceutical companies asking if and how they could help. When I pointed out to them that what they were being asked to do was to produce a new drug for a rare complication of a rare disease with very limited sales; that they would need to go through the official toxicity testing, clinical trials and obtain a product license, not surprisingly, they soon lost interest. Even in those days the cost of introducing a new drug was enormous and as pharmaceutical companies must make a profit on their investment to stay in business their reluctance to be involved was understandable. Clearly there would be little or no financial advantage should the venture prove a therapeutic success and there was much to be lost if any mishap should befall. It seems probable that the share holders would not be too happy should the company found itself involved in litigation. A number of small chemical companies also made enquiries with the same result except for Cambrian Chemicals who, although they backed off at this juncture, retained an interest which eventually bore fruit.

It would appear that my letter had not had the desired effect. The venture had come to naught. Other tactics were required so, in 1976, under the guise that this was the 21st birthday of penicillamine, I convened a scientific meeting held at my old undergraduate college in Cambridge, Trinity Hall. This was the meeting, referred to earlier, sponsored by Dista Products, thanks to the good will of their medical director, Dr. Hugh Lyle. Although the title of the meeting was 'Penicillamine at 21' the real topic under discussion was 'Drugs for Rare Diseases'. I managed to persuade both the Department of Health and also the pharmaceutical industry to send representatives; also the malpractice insurance societies, an expert in medical ethics and a number of interested physicians, the press were also invited. The general tone of the meeting was sympathetic to my problem. It was felt that those factors inhibiting research and development in the field of non-profit making drugs were fear of litigation,fear of damages and perhaps, worst of all fear of the loss of good name and pillorying by the news media should any unexpected toxic reaction occur. The consensus was that a solution could be found if the Department of Health itself would take out a product license for the compound in question. The manufacturer would then simply be responsible for supplying the required chemical to government specification. Purity would be tested by the laboratory of the Government Chemist and the Department of Health would be responsible for any further toxicity testing and side effects. Clearly no pharmaceutical company would be prepared to take on all these responsibilities on the request of a single research worker. To my surprise this meeting had thus resulted in significant progress, even if it took many years to mature. Government departments have a genius all of their own for procrastination and the Department of Health proved to be no exception. However it is quite remarkable that they allowed themselves to be involved in this unlikely undertaking. It might have been that my cynicism was, after all, ill founded.

The first tangible benefit was that The Government Chemist undertook not only to test the purity of our final product but also to examine the source material for impurities and to determine the specifications to be met for the drug to be officially adopted. A further huge advance was the fact that, thanks to Mr. Graham Tucker, Cambrian Chemicals came back and offered to manufacture trientine to the required specifications. Here I have to make specific thanks to two other members of the team at Cambrian Chemicals, Roger Humphries who made liaison with me to ascertained the nature of my requirements and made the necessary arrangements and to Rupert Purchase, their chief chemist, who worked out a method of purification, based on Hal Dixon's original work, that could be used on a commercial scale. He was also able to isolate three major impurities from the technical grade source material which enabled these three compounds to be used as chromatographic standards for the analysis of trientine. Both have remained good friends ever since and Rupert is regularly attends and contributes to the annual meeting of the Wilson's disease Support Group. In return for these advances I undertook to supply the Department of Health with clinical data on the patients treated and to keep them up to date on future developments and any possible toxic reactions. My contact here was John Sloggem who played a major role in securing the future supply of trientine. The work of production and encapsulation of trientine was later taken over by K&K-Greeff and then Univar. This has ensured a reliable supply of the drug for the past 30 years. This was indeed an enormous advance and one which I could have nor reasonably expected when I set up the Trinity Hall meeting.

While all these negotiations were in progress over several years the situation in the clinic did not stand still. Clinical situations never do and patients have a way of forcing a sense of urgency on their doctors which it seemed quite impossible to convey to the bureaucrats in the Department of Health whose motto appears to be safety first, progress must follow later. Two further patients presented themselves. Jill, a teenage girl was referred by her very astute general practitioner. She had just lost her elder sister who had clearly died of undiagnosed Wilson disease at St Elsewhere's Hospital in London. Jill, who had the very earliest symptoms of neurological damage, rapidly developed penicillamine toxicity and needed changing to trientine. The second, also a young woman, was a foreign student from Iran. studying at an English language school in Cambridge. She also needed changing from penicillamine to trientine. The problem here was that she was due soon to return home and this would commit us to sending her capsules, on a regular and perhaps indefinite basis, to Iran; a commitment I had previously decided could not be sustainable. When the time came we did indeed bite the bullet and make the necessary dispatches, though how the local customs officers would view the parcels I could only guess. Eventually the problem was unexpectedly solved by this patient migrating to the United States whence I referred her to my counterpart in that country, Herb Scheinberg. If I thought that I had overcome all current problems I was soon to be disillusioned. The reaction Jill had developed to penicillamine was soon reactivated by trientine. How this new and entirely unexpected life threatening situation was dealt with I will consider later. Shortly after this a girl from Egypt was referred from that Mecca of neurological disease, The National Hospital, Queen Square, for treatment with trientine. This presented no clinical difficulties in making the change but again raised the spectre of mailing the drug overseas pending the possibility of the patients parents being able to make arrangements, on return home, for some official recognition of the supply problem. For a while this worked well but did, eventually, break down, but that is another story. During 1978 there was a continued steady stream of patients referred for this new medication, Sardinia proving one of the most fruitful sources. Presumably the gene had spread through a small island population which had remained relatively inbred and stable until the advent of the tourist trade. Being the progenitor and sole supplier of trientine certainly had its benefits in keeping my clinic at the forefront of Wilson disease research and management but did increase the work load as scarcely any patient, once on the books, was ever lost to follow up. The results of treatment, particularly in the disappearance of most or all of their neurological disability, made it all a most rewarding exercise. Mean time negotiations with the Ministry dragged on, in all for a period of nine years. They were clearly sympathetic to my particular problem and anxious to help, but, in their view, there was no case for precipitate action.

However, compared with the major political and financial problems facing the Minister this was only a minor consideration. I may be unjust in my thinking but I suspected that, being a minor problem, it was given to a minor official to deal with. But if he, or she, made the wrong decision it would clearly jeopardise future chances of promotion so it must be safer to keep the ball in play until the time came for transfer to another post The problem could then be safely handed on to a successor who would then have to make a decision, or keep the ball in play for as long as possible. To follow this strategy it was necessary for them that I maintain a flow of data so that they could pass this on to those further up the echelon. Thus I was asked for regular up dates on the clinical situation and the response of patients to treatment. It seemed rather like the children's game of passing the parcel, the one holding the parcel when the music stops being the loser. From the Ministry's point of view this was a remarkably successful strategy. After several years I was no further forward in getting the promised product license. On the other side of the Atlantic the orphan drug lobby had become active in the United States and had even spawned a television programme and the book 'Orphan Drugs' edited by Fred Karch, to which I have referred earlier. This, in turn, led to action in Congress in the early 1980s and I was visited by Congressman Waxman who was active in promoting the Orphan Drugs Act. I do not know whether he learned anything useful from this visit but it was a pleasure to take him to see the home of George Washington's ancestors, at Sulgrave Manor in Northamptonshire. Not wanting to be beaten to legalization of my drug by the US I increased pressure on the Ministry and, with the cooperation of Herb Scheinberg organised a small international meeting on Orphan Drugs and Orphan Diseases at Leeds castle in Kent in the autumn of 1985, under the sponsorship of the Fulbright Commission. To my delight, shortly before the meeting assembled, the Ministry issued a limited product license, trientine could be used only for Wilson's disease patients who had proved intolerant to penicillamine. Whilst this meeting was basically scientific I had invited the Rev. Gordon Dunstan to come and advise us on the medical ethics involved, a subject in which he was the acknowledged expert. Ethics must always be considered in the introduction of new drugs for patients with rare diseases, drugs which, of the very nature of the situation, can not go through the extensive testing that drugs introduced by industry, for common diseases, needs must undergo.

One point I raised, which was troubling me, was this, what is the responsibility of a physician who wishes to invest in an expensive procedure, for the benefit of a single patient, if this might lead to constraints on treatments available to the larger community. Personally I believed the duty of the doctor was to his individual patient but I could see that the official in charge of the budget would think otherwise. In this situation the position of the doctor and the budget holder are mutually incompatible. After only a brief consideration Gordon Dunstan gave me the answer I was hoping for, '*The duty of the individual doctor was to his patient and not to the community*'. Some short while after this meeting the FDA also issued a product license for the use of trientine in the USA, this time we had beaten our American cousins in the race for legitimacy. It really was a triumph that a new drug, originally designed for a single patient with a rare complication in the management of a rare disease had got official recognition in both the UK and the USA.

Another interesting story of the 1970 was of a pair of identical twins referred by their general practitioner with an apologetic letter saying he was afraid he was wasting my time but that their mother insisted that I should see them. The story was that an elder brother had died, a few years earlier in a specialist children's hospital in London of undiagnosed liver disease. When one of the twins developed similar symptoms mother remembered having read an article in Reader's Digest about Wilson's disease and she was convinced that this is what her children had. The general practitioner had first referred the twins to London where the report said there was no evidence of Wilson's disease. But mother insisted that this must be wrong, so the twins ended up in Cambridge. The twin who first showed signs had been treated with steroids and showed many of the unwanted side effects of this drug. Simple laboratory tests soon proved that mother was right and both twins, as genetics dictated, did indeed have Wilson's disease. I immediately stopped the steroids and started them on penicillamine. They have never looked back and are so alike I can not tell one from the other. I was so intrigued by this story of mother making the diagnosis from Reader's Digest that I told it to my friend Herb Scheinberg whose immediate response was, yes he had himself written that article. It truly is a small world. I was impressed by mother's determination to get the correct diagnosis in the face of all the odds. I have found, as in other families, that mothers are much more persistent than fathers in this respect! One policy which I have always followed was to test all children of a Wilson disease parent to see if any such child is at risk of developing the disease. Any child must, by definition, carry one abnormal gene inherited from the affected parent. The chance of such a parent marrying a carrier is now estimated at approximately 1/90 and of the second parent passing on this gene is 1/2 so the risk to an infant is of the order of 1/180; not a great risk In 50 years of study of Wilson disease I detected one new born who had inherited the two abnormal genes for Wilson's disease. He was put on prophylactic treatment at the age of 2 years and has subsequently developed normally with no sign of the disease making its unwelcome appearance.

I must now take a step back to the spring of 1955 when I became involved in patients with Wilson disease. Little was known about the disease at that time. It can briefly be summarized as follows: it was a disease of youngsters in which damage occurred in those regions of the brain controlling movement; there were visible deposits of copper in cornea of the eyes known as Kayser Fleischer rings (Fig. **7**) there was an associated scarring of the liver; there was an excess of copper in the brain and the liver; there was excess copper in the urine, but accompanied by subnormal amounts of copper and the copper carrying protein in the blood; that the kidneys leaked certain small molecules such as sugars, aminoacids and calcium; temporary improvement could be achieved by treatment with the cooper binding drug BAL; the disease was also known to be inherited, one gene from each parent. An alternative school of thought, led by Uzman and Denny Brown, believed that the disease was one of protein or peptide metabolism and that copper deposition in the tissues was merely a secondary phenomenon of little relevance to the progress of the disease; they further claimed that abnormal peptides could be found in the urine to support their claim.

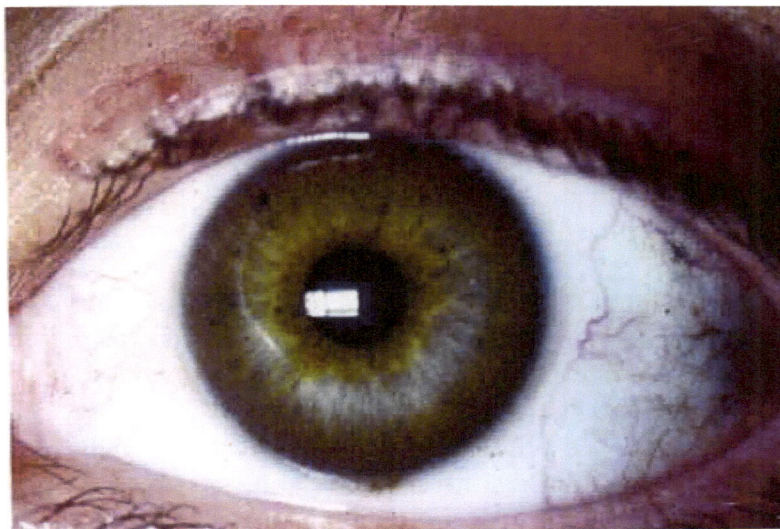

Fig. (7). The eye of a patient with newly diagnosed Wilson's disease showing the brown deposit of copper surrounding the iris. This is known as the Kayser Fleischer ring. It will disappear with copper removing treatment.

What I needed to establish was what would happen, in the long run, to a patient when he or she was started on highly effective copper removing treatment with D-penicillamine. This was, of course, quite unknown and I would be moving into new and uncharted territory. That meant everything had to be carefully assessed and documented meticulously, both the patients clinical response, hopefully improvement in movement control and improvement in signs of liver damage. Also I needed to record all changes in their biochemistry, for better or for worse: hopefully a lowering of the blood and urine copper levels and improvement in liver function and in kidney function, and also any possible changes in the blood count. To this effect I devised a routine whereby patients were admitted to Addenbrooke's Hospital on a Sunday or Monday, a standard set of tests were run through during the week, any necessary steps taken to sort out any other problems that the patient might have and allow them home for the following weekend. This was the optimum arrangement both for assessing progress and reducing time in hospital to a minimum. It had one great drawback. My allocated beds were empty on Saturday and Sunday so that any emergency admission to the hospital might fill the vacancy and leave no bed for my next Monday morning patient. What I needed was a model patient to be slipped into the bed to keep it free for my next admission.! Such would have been a great help. All new patients, invariably referred from considerable distances in this country or from abroad, were kept as long as was necessary for establishing the basal biochemical parameters which were essential for future reference, tape recording any speech defects and, on occasions filming movement disorders. Then determining whether penicillamine or trientine would give the best copper excretion before making them ready and able to return home. Timing of the follow up necessarily depended on how far away the patient lived but it was my endeavour to see everyone, where possible, at least once a year or more often if necessary. Though this could not always be achieved it did set a standard and most patients ended up by becoming not only regular in attendance but also friends and it was always my object to help with their social problems, where possible, as well as the medical ones although the former were usually more difficult to solve. Dr Gerald Stern actually suggested, surely in jest, that I knew so much about my patients that I could complete their income tax returns! Would that I could do my own.

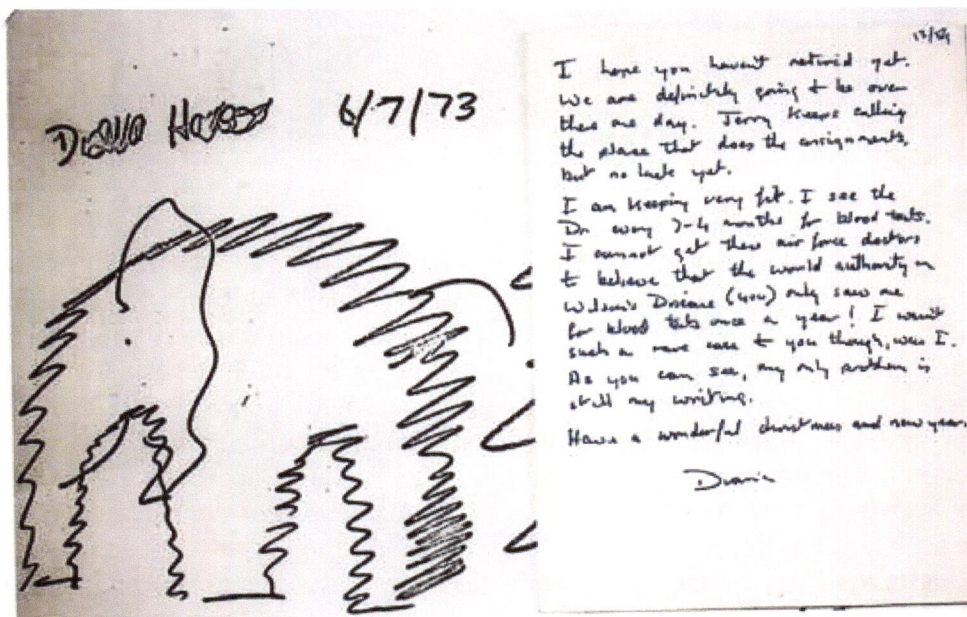

Fig. (8). Another example of improvement in handwriting can be achieved by the treatment of patients with Wilson's disease with penicillamine the 1973 effort shows a standard 'Walshe elephant' clearly illustrating severe tremor. The handwriting is of 11 years later after she married and emigrated to the USA.

Experience showed that the best method of assessing a patient's clinical progress was simply to sit and talk with them and watch their movements and their response to questions. I found it mattered little to the patient if they had lost their knee jerks, it did matter if they could not bend down and tie up a shoe lace or complete other simple tasks that we all take for granted. However such unsupported statements would not convince my colleagues, definitive evidence had to be documented. The easiest way to show control of movement is to ask the patient to write down his name and date, to this I added a simple drawing, now known as the standard Walshe Elephant. (Fig. **8**) A rather more sophisticated technique was to fix a small light to each hand and, in a darkened room, to ask the patient to hold a given posture or make certain specific movements for a standard time in front of an exposed photographic plate, any tremor or involuntary movement would then be shown by movements of the lights, green for the right hand, red for the left. These procedures were both cheap and easy to perform and by repeating them on each visit progress was easily recorded (Fig. **9**). Sometimes video films were also made and tape recordings of any speech defect. As patients improved they often forgot how disabled they had been and showing them this evidence gave great encouragement even when progress was slow. Eventually the great majority of patients have been able to return to a normal standard of living although, unfortunately, a small number have remained more or less disabled.

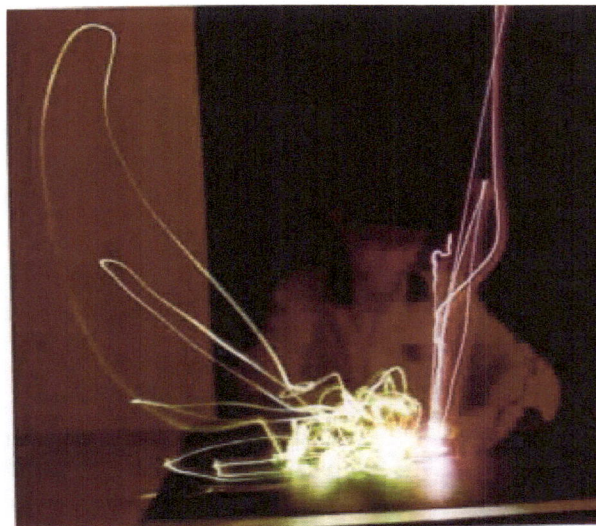

Fig. (9). Abnormal ballistic movement recorded by finger lights. The patient was asked to place six matches in a box in 30 seconds

The response to treatment of a new patient I could never predict, all I could say was that the great majority would respond well but a very small percentage unfortunately did not do so The standard biochemical tests and brain scans gave no clue as to this, after nigh on 50 years experience, an accurate prediction still eluded me. As far as laboratory tests were concerned it was necessary to determine if abnormal liver function would improve, if kidney function could be improved and what would happen to the abnormalities of the blood and urine copper levels recorded on first admission. Would the blood copper level approach the normal value or would it drop even further, what would happen to the serum copper carrying protein caeruloplasmin and what would happen to the abnormal amounts of copper present in the liver which had taken many years to accumulate. Also it was necessary to document any changes that occurred to the amount of copper excreted in the urine; would this decrease give an accurate reflection of a lessening of the body stores of the metal?

Around 1970 it became apparent that I needed to know more about the dynamics of penicillamine, How fast and how completely was it absorbed from the gut. What was its distribution in the body. Was the molecule broken down or otherwise modified by the liver. How was it excreted.? Looking back it seems remarkable that this compound had been officially recognized and entered into the pharmacopoeia without any effort on my part, or that of any other worker in this field, to document these basic facts. The easiest way to obtain this information was to get the molecule labeled with a radioactive tracer so that it could be readily detected at very low concentrations in body fluids. With the help of a grant from the Medical Research Council I enlisted the help of Dr. J.R. Ogle of the Radiochemical Centre at Amersham to prepare for me a batch of penicillamine labeled on the sulphur atom. Thus it was possible to show that penicillamine was rapidly absorbed from the gut and reached a peak concentration in the plasma in two to five hours, after which it was equally rapidly cleared by the kidneys but that traces could still be detected in the plasma up to 48 hours bound to other plasma proteins. The molecule was not broken down in the liver, much was excreted unchanged, but some was conjugated to other small molecules. One question was answered, penicillamine was not in any way handled differently by the two patients who had shown an unfavouable reaction to its administration. Presumably it was the formation of penicillamine protein complexes that led to the development of an immune complex reaction in susceptible individuals.

By the time the application for a product license for trientine had arrived such basic information was essential. Trientine is not an easy compound to identify in biological systems chemically so that the same approach of detection by radiochemical assay was necessary.Again the Medical Research Council provided the necessary financial help and the Radiochemical Centre at Amersham prepared the labelled trientine for me, this time the label was on all the carbon atoms in the molecule. As we had only small amounts of the compound the studies were carried out on rats. This had the advantage that it was possible to assay a variety of body tissues for radioactivity and make a detailed picture of distribution in the body. These studies showed that the drug was very poorly absorbed from the gut, only about twenty percent of the dose. It could be detected in all body tissues, principally in the kidneys where it was concentrated for excretion in the urine. Again we were able to show that it was not broken down in the body but excreted conjugated to other small molecules It was also possible to show that, contrary to my expectation, the molecule could be shown to have passed through the cell membrane and it could certainly be detected in the cells by exposing a radiosensitive film on microscope sections of liver. I was left to speculate that if trientine had such a powerful action in promoting copper excretion when given by mouth, when only a small percentage of the dose was absorbed, how active it might be if given by vein. I never had the courage to carry out this experiment in man. As data accumulated over the years it became apparent that continued treatment with this drug was not associated with any serious toxicity, but a very few patients did develop some gastrointestinal problems and that pregnancy presented no greater risk than in the normal. Meanwhile the great majority of patients improved to a remarkable extent from both the hepatic and neurological lesions. The results of biochemical tests were also encouraging. The concentration of copper in the blood fell, the amount of the metal excreted in the urine dropped, often back to the normal. There were those who suggested that this was due to treatment losing its efficacy, whereas it was, in practice, due to depletion of the abnormal body stores of the metal. Simply there was less to be mobilized. Further proof of benefit was to be seen in the disappearance of the copper deposits in the eyes and, as I was able to show much later, a reduction in the excess copper deposits in the liver. In fact our studies with radiocopper showed that the pattern of copper uptake by the liver returned to the presymptomatic pattern after prolonged treatment.

Thus by the early 1980s this whole venture appeared to be a significant success story. A hitherto fatal disease of young people had been turned into one in which most patients could reasonably expect to make a useful recovery. However it had to be admitted that a very small number did not respond to treatment, some remaining stuck with varying degrees of disability and a very few indeed, as I remember four out of over three hundred patients, went steadily down hill and died despite my very best efforts to reverse their steady decline. I never knew why, despite my very best efforts, this happened; possibly it was due to a very unfavourable gene mutation, but with almost 300 mutations now identified, and most patients having two different mutations, the possible permutations and combinations available means that this hypothesis will be very difficult to prove. Recovery in most cases is slow, after all it had taken the majority of patients, when first seen, some ten to twenty years to accumulate toxic concentrations of copper and these can not be mobilized and removed overnight. Usually it took from six months to a year before useful return of function occurred. Very occasionally improvement took place remarkably quickly; I remember particularly the case of a young woman of 18 years who was referred from Athens with a two year history of deteriorating health. Her most notable problem was a change in her speech and a slowing down of all her movements. Wilson disease was diagnosed and treatment with penicillamine was started. Over the next three months she became somewhat more disabled and hence referred to my clinic. My investigations confirmed the diagnosis and her CAT brain scan showed large cavities in the motor ganglia of the brain suggesting a very poor prognosis. I added trientine to her treatment regime. After two weeks she started to improve and I returned her to her doctor in Athens. All went well for a further two months then she deteriorated rapidly and when she came back to me, three months after I had discharged her, she appeared to be in the final stage of her illness, incapable of any coordinated movement, unable to speak or swallow. Indeed the driver who brought her up from London airport said he thought she would die on the journey and said he would never transport another patient for me ! My immediate finding was that this patient had become grossly anaemic and after the anaemia was corrected by a blood transfusion she started to make a rapid improvement. Some years later I saw another patient in whom the development of anaemia also resulted in a great increase in the neurological lesions of Wilson disease. Clearly anaemia is something which must be avoided in these cases. After only three weeks my Greek patient was able to return home and only a year later she was able to show me around the acropolis in Athens (Fig. **10).** Following her second admission she had made one of the most rapid recoveries I had ever seen. She also made a first in whom it was possible to show that the brain cavities, demonstrated on her first admission, appeared to heal completely as demonstrated by later scanning, hereby suggesting that recovery of lost neurones in the brain was indeed a possibility, despite the official doctrine that this could never take place.

At some time in the 1980s Professor Weatherall, Nuffield Professor of Medicine in Oxford, contacted me to see if I could supply him with DNA from my Wilson disease patients as he hoped to be able to clone the gene. As my studies with Ruth Sanger on possible blood group linkages had yielded nothing I was only too happy to cooperate. I regularly sent him samples and he was able to set up a number of immortal cell lines from these. Later, to my great disappointment, he abandoned this line of research. However the work was not wasted as all the samples were sent on to Professor Diane Wilson Cox in Toronto. Diane was, and still is, a distinguished geneticist who was also working on the Wilson disease gene. Thus I continued to send DNA, but to Toronto rather than Oxford. I felt rewarded when Diane published her findings, the identification of the mutant gene as a copper transporting P-type ATPase, ATPase 7b, which controlled the movement the metal through cell walls. This important publication appeared in the journal Nature at the same time a similar identifications by two other groups of workers. It was indeed a triple first. Since then, up to my retirement, I continued to send samples and this helped in the identification of nearly three hundred different pathological mutations.

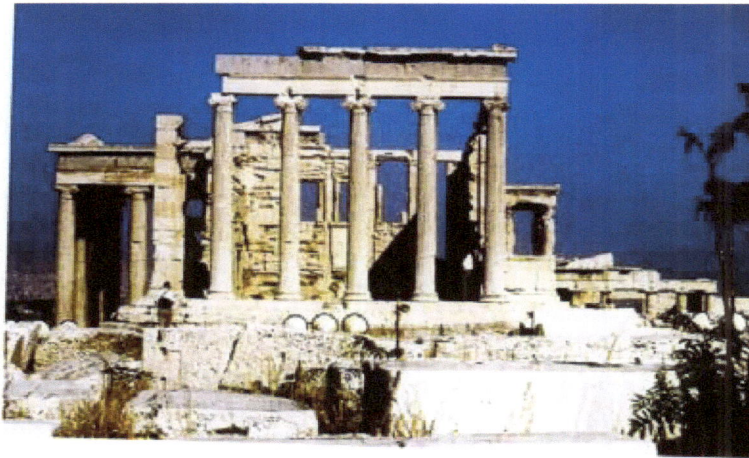

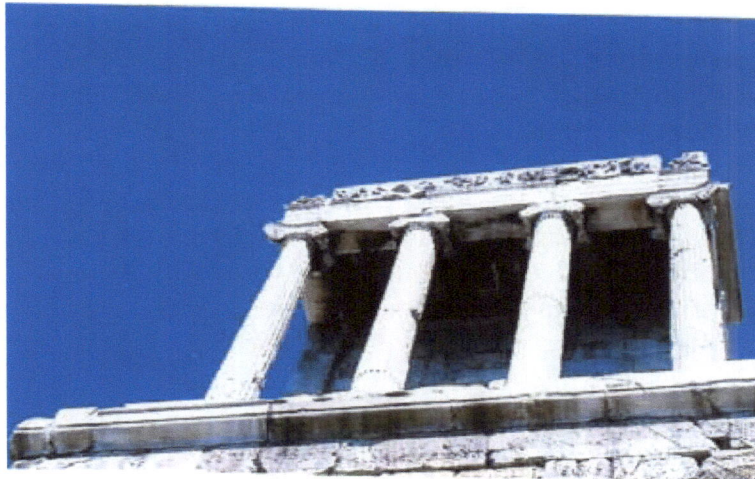

Fig. (10). The Athenian acropolis where I met one of my Greek Patients fifteen months after she had been admitted to Addenrooke's Hospital, apparently in the terminal stage of Wilson's disease, incapable of any coordinated movement. At this time she was training as a English Language Teacher. Illustrated here Are the temples of Erectheus and Apteros Nike (Wingless Vicory).

This discovery together with the basic work on the role of copper in Wilson's disease has led directly to a much greater understanding in the biochemistry of copper-trafficking proteins. There have been no significant additions to our knowledge of Wilson disease since that date. It is to be hoped that eventually this work may lead to a better understanding of why a small number of patients still fail to respond to treatment.

CHAPTER 6

Going International and yet more Problems

Away! Away! For I will fly to thee
Keats, Ode to a Nightingale.

Abstract: Inevitably the news of the success of penicillamine treatment for patients with Wilson's disease spread and calls came from abroad for help. My first overseas call for help came from Rheims, then Vienna and the last one was from Rome. Unfortunately I was not able to help any of these patients as they were already on penicillamine and had failed to respond and no other therapies were available at the time of those visits although the patient from Vienna was eventually transferred to Cambridge. However the television programme on the BBC Overseas Service did result in the opening of a flood gate of patients from Europe and then the Middle East. The first of these patients came from Hungary and this was closely followed by patients from Italy, including Sardinia, Spain, Yugoslavia (as was), Greece, Turkey, Iran, Iraq, The Yemen and Egypt. There was also one each from the USA and South Africa.
A new problem arose with a home patient who developed intolerance to penicillamine, trientne BAL and zinc treatment. A new drug had to be found for her. Earlier workers had investigated the use of molybdate on good theoretical basis but had used the wrong salt. This problem was solved by using a sulphur molybdate compound which was known to induce copper deficiency in sheep. As nothing was known of its safety in many I successfully assayed this first on myself.

Inevitably, as the news of the success of penicillamine treatment spread abroad, probably at least in part, as a result of the overseas BBC television programme, I received a number of request to see patients in their own countries. Some of these were referred by the doctors, some came by the enterprise of the patients themselves. The first such call was to a small boy in Reims. I flew to Paris and then took a train to Reims where the paeditrician in charge, Dr Fandre, met me and took me to the hospital to see his patient with an advanced stage of Wilson disease He was already taking penicillamine and had not responded to treatment. At that time there was no other available treatment and there was little I could do to help except suggest some methods of reducing the absorption of copper from the diet. I never heard if this helped but I think it unlikely. However I took the opportunity to visit the cathedral and also the abbey church of St Remi, which in some ways I found more interesting. It has some splendid early stained glass which, many years later, I was able to photograph. I kept contact with Dr Fandre and only last year had the honour to be invited to his grand daughter's wedding. Unfortunately I was forced to decline as my wife and I had come to the end of our traveling days. I had similarly, again with great regret, to decline an invitation to the wedding of a colleague in Salonika.A Greek Orthodox wedding would have been a great experience.

The next overseas call was to Vienna. I already knew this patient's doctor and I had every confidence that he was giving the best possible treatment. When I arrived I found a young man, the only child of devoted parents, with gross postural deformities from muscular spasms. He was being nursed in a very over crowded ward which I though far from ideal. But, as with the boy in Rheims, there was no other treatment but penicillamine available at the time and there was little I could do to help. The parents were most anxious that I would take their son back to Cambridge but I tried to explain to them that this would be a very expensive exercise for them and that I did not think it would help. I returned home empty handed. However mothers never give up and the parents continued to pressurize me to take their son. Eventually, against my better judgment, I agreed and Axel was duly admitted to the old Addenbrooke's Hospital. At that time I had the good fortune to have an exceptionally efficient ward sister. In the 1960s nursing was still taught as an apprenticeship not as an academic discipline so that standards of personal care were much higher than they are today.

By dint of diligent nursing techniques the giant bed sore with which Axel arrived was cured and this was the only benefit it was possible to give him. It did cause some friction for mother, who sat at the end of the bed watching everything with a gimlet like gaze, and she did not like seeing her son turned every half hour and kept turning him back onto the bed sore. Sister would immediately turn him again to which mother strongly objected; I had to act as a peace maker between the two. The question arose as to whether Axel should have neurosurgery to reduce his spasms and mother was keen on this line of approach. I therefore made the necessary arrangements and he was transferred to the appropriate surgical ward. Surgery was carried out the following day and when I visited him a couple of days later it was apparent to me, though not apparently to the surgical team, that Axel had developed pneumonia. I felt that as there was no realistic possibility of any useful recovery I should take no action. As I had anticipated Axel eventually died of this complication and his body was flown back to Vienna with his grieving mother.

At some stage there was a call to Switzerland, but apart from the episode when I successfully took a blood sample from a very small child, to the surprise of his Swiss doctor who had always had great trouble with this manoeuvre, I have no recollection of the visit. Finally there was a call to Rome. Looking at the possible travel arrangements I decided that if I caught an early flight the whole exercise could be completed in a day. This meant spending the night in one of the hotels situated adjacent to London Air Port. I motored down to Heath row and on reaching the last roundabout before entering the air port I saw my hotel on the right. I took the slip road towards it only to find myself back on the motorway heading west. Unworried by this I immediately took the turning off on to the M25, the London orbital motorway, thinking that I could cross over the west bound M4 and rejoin it going east back to Heath Row. Unfortunately for me there was no slip road allowing this manoeuvre and I had to travel for about 20 miles before I could turn and make my way back to my hotel! I caught the first flight the next morning and arriving at the hospital in Rome I again found the situation was unsatisfactory. The patients illness was far advanced and, in addition, the ward overcrowded. I made some suggestions but without too much hope that they would help. After the consultation the physician asked me what I would like to see in Rome and, having been there before, I opted for Hadrian's villa which I had not been able to include in my previous visit. I never heard the final outcome of this case but the prognosis did not look at all good. I was driven back to the airport by Massimo, my first Italian patient. I thought this a striking proof of his recovery that he was able to negotiate a car safely through the undisciplined chaos of Rome's traffic. I also saw some patients on several occasions when attending conferences abroad and, on one occasion, when visiting Sardinia with a view to organizing a conference in that island I was able to follow up on patients I had seen in Cambridge previously. Sardinia seemed to me to be a suitable place for such a meeting as the gene is clearly relatively common there and several patients had been referred to me from that island.. Nothing came of the proposed conference in that location, the meeting was finally held in the superb surroundings of Leeds Castle.

The situation with patients who came from abroad to see me in Cambridge, and later in London, was very much more satisfactory. The great majority benefiting from their visits. The first such patient was a young girl from Hungary. She arrived in 1963 after an unsuccessful stop off in Switzerland. She made an excellent recovery and later went to University in Vienna to study mathematics. She remained on my follow up books until I retired, but we still keep in contact by letter. The last time I saw her was, when attending a conference in Vienna, I was invited to her home and met her two charming daughters. After my programme on the BBC overseas service there was a steady flow of patients from Europe and, later, the Middle

East. The next to come was Massimo from Rome and after that the flood gates opened and about one third of all my new patients came from abroad. A few from the major countries of Western Europe, France, Germany, Holland, Spain and Portugal, more from central Europe, Czechoslovakia, Hungary and Poland. Many more from around the Mediterranean basin, Italy, Greece, Yugoslavia (as was), Turkey and even Iraq, Iran, the Yemen and Egypt. In addition there was one each from the USA and South Africa. The South African patient I handled rather differently from all the others. The rate of exchange between Rand and the pound was so unfavourable that the financial burden to this young man's parents was such that I tried to save them money as far as possible. I therefore did not see the patient in my clinic, which would have cost him a fee to the hospital, I think about that time of around £100. Therefore, to save his parents this expense, I saw him in his hotel. He was very severely disabled by muscular spasms, and difficulty with speech and swallowing. How he managed on the long flight from South Africa I can not think. It must have been a nightmare for his mother and an ordeal for the patient, much less the cabin staff. He had been treated, quite reasonably, with penicillamine but had failed completely to show any benefit. Clearly something had to be done and under the limited circumstances it was difficult to know what. The only possibility, and this did not give much hope, was to try changing his treatment to trientine. I arranged for his mother to pick up enough to keep him going till they returned home and set up a local supply. I must admit it was to my surprise that the change apparently worked remarkably well and the patient made a complete recovery. However, there has been a continuing difficulty in obtaining trientine in South Africa and the steady fall n the value of the Rand has increased the problem. At one time I even suggested to his parents that, as they were of Italian extraction, they should move to that country where his medication would be ensured. They have not yet found it necessary to take that step but the problem remains and a satisfactory solution has yet to be found. Other patients in that unhappy country are also involved and I worry for them too. The uncertain political future for South Africa does not suggest to me that the prognosis is good. But in a country in which the spread of AIDS is a major health problem the fate of a few patients with Wilson's disease is not likely to cut much ice.

Whilst all this was going on the care of home patients continued unabated and, inevitably, new problems arose. Charles Dickens, in' Our Mutual Friend', wrote, '*Mr. Podsnap.....even acquired a peculiar flourish of his right arm in often clearing the world of its most difficult problems, by sweeping them behind him'*. Unfortunately clinical problems can not be so easily solved as by sweeping them away. In the early 1980s a small number of patients were seen who had either not responded well to standard treatment or who had developed reactions to both penicillamine and trientine. The most worrying of these was Jill, who has already been mentioned, and whose earlier misadventures had left her with serious kidney damage. I therefore started her on zinc sulphate in order to block any further absorption of copper from her diet. After a year she remained in a stable condition but said that the abdominal pain this treatment caused her was such that she would rather die than continue with it. A biopsy of her liver at that time showed that there had been an alarmingly increase in the concentration of copper during her time on zinc and there was also much cellular damage. I therefore decided to try BAL. Jill had such a severe reaction to a single dose that further treatment with this drug was clearly not an option. This presented me with the same problem that Robert had done ten years before, to take no action must inevitably result in Jill's death. I remembered that some years earlier a colleague, I would like to give him due credit but I have no note of who this was, suggested that a salt of molybdenum, a metallic element, might be of use in counteracting the toxic action of copper.

The rationale of this idea was the observation, well known to the veterinary profession, that sheep that grazed on pastures contaminated with this metal and rich in sulphur gave birth to lambs with abnormalities of the nervous system, known as sway back, associated with a deficiency of copper. As long ago as the early 1950s a team of doctors in Birmingham had tried to use the oxide of molybdenum to treat Wilson disease patients with out success so what was the point of trying again ? Well there was a point; the Birmingham team had not realized that there is a great difference in the digestive processes between man and sheep ! Sheep are ruminants and the molybdate ingested from the sulphur rich pasture was converted in the abomasums (the fourth stomach) of the sheep to a compound known as tetrathio molybdate and it is this compound that has a very powerful anticopper action. Humans, not being ruminants and not having four stomachs, are unable to effect this conversion and since molybdate itself has no anticopper action the use of this particular compound inevitably led to the failure of this therapy in the Birmingham trial. I therefore decided that, if I could obtain some pure tetrathio molybdate, it would be well worth having another look. Here again I was exceptionally lucky, an inorganic biochemist in Leicester, Stuart Laurie, very kindly agreed to synthesise some tetrathio molybdate for me as the ammonium salt. As nothing was known about its toxicity in man, as with my earlier introduction of penicillamine, there was nothing to do but take it myself first to assess its safety. This I did for a week with out ill effect, but the experiment did yield some interesting biochemical findings which were encouraging. The evidence suggested that the copper in the blood became much more tightly bound to a molybdate-protein complex but that there was little or no effect on the amount of copper excreted in the urine. In Jill however, to my surprise, there was a great increase in the amount of copper in the serum and a very modest increase in the urine copper after taking a test dose of ammonium tetrathiomolybdate. Further studies in other patients supported my theory that the copper in the serum was very much more tightly bound to protein than before this treatment. When I gave both radioactive copper and molybdate to patients it showed that this completely blocked the absorption of the metal from the gut and was even more effective in this respect than zinc salts.

I next obtained a small quantity of radiolabelled ammonium tetrathiomolybdate which was fed to rats. These studies showed that the compound was readily absorbed from the gut and was detectable in most body tissues. It was also rapidly cleared by the kidneys. A new treatment had become available to supplement penicillamine and trientine and it appeared to be superior to zinc in blocking copper absorption from the gut. It also had the additional advantage of binding the copper already present in the body so tightly that it became metabolically inert. Despite the difficulty in obtaining supplies it has proved subsequently to be of benefit to a small number of patients. These findings were presented at the conference held at Leeds Castle in 1985 but following my retirement from Cambridge my part time post in London made it impossible for me to pursue this line of research further. Later, however, tetrathio molybdate for a treatment for Wilson's disease has been enthusiastically adopted by Dr. Brewer in the USA. where he is hoping to obtain official backing from the FDA for its use and also a reliable commercial supply of the compound. The problem has remained, in this country, of obtaining a regular supply and a product license. For about ten years of the initial studies Dr. Laurie generously continued to synthesise and supply me with thiomolybdate but he has now retired and the compound is no longer available for use in this country. Dr Rupert Purchase, who solved the problem of commercial trientine production, has volunteered to synthesise tetrathio molybdate at the required purity but, at the time of writing it has proved impossible to obtain any official backing and until someone is prepared to put their head on the block and says go ahead the difficulty of future supplies and the official acceptance of this line of treatment remains unsolved. Since I am now retired, I am, unfortunately, no longer in a position to apply pressure on either the Department of Health, NICE or the medical malpractice insurance companies who will need to be prepared to underwrite any doctor brave enough to use this therapy.

By 1985 I had reached the official retirement age for NHS doctors but, being a University employed honorary physician I had a further two years to go, the University retiring age, at that time was 67 years: this meant I had time to look for some future, long term arrangements for my patients. Meanwhile the routine care of patients continued and all three of the therapies I had introduced found their use, though thiomolybdate was reserved for only a very small number of patients. In one of these patients it actually damaged her bone marrow necessitating instant withdrawal. Fortunately her marrow rapidly recovered, but this observation meant that all future patients on this drug need to have their blood counts closely monitored at least for the first few months of treatment. By the summer of 1987 I was seriously worried about future arrangements for this very large number of Wilson disease patients that I had cared for, some for many years. Jill was of particular concern. I realized that no one would be prepared to take the medicolegal risk of continuing with unlicensed tetrathiomolybdate. As her parents had moved from Essex to Cambridge to be near the Hospital I felt it would be safe to try and re-establish treatment with trientine by using a minimal dose and watching her renal function on a regular basis for signs of recurrent damage. Earlier Jill had had a rather unexpected problem, she had attended the hospital New Year's eve party when, whilst dancing, she was seized by severe abdominal pain and collapsed. She was taken to the accident department where she was told to take an indigestion medicine and go home to bed. Two days later her mother rang me to say that Jill was still very poorly and what should she do. I said put her in a taxi and bring her straight to my ward. Examination confirmed my suspicion that she had suffered an intraperitoneal bleed which scanning showed to have come from a rupture of the splenic artery which required immediate surgery. I know that New Year's eve diagnoses can be difficult but I thought this was a bad error on the part of the accident and emergency team. Fortunately Jill survived with out any long term complications from this incident.

Another problem that presented itself in my last year at Addenbrookes Hospital was that of a 13 year old lad, Mark, from Norfolk, who was referred with a severe neurological lesion. He was obviously going to be in hospital for some time. Unfortunately he proved to be one of those rare but unfortunate patients who failed to respond to any of the treatments available. Although his disease was stabilized he remained in need of a lot of help with his normal day to day activities. However it proved impossible to return him home; his parents were separated and neither was prepared to have him back. A long stay in hospital is anything but desirable for a teenage boy. There was an arrangement where by such children did receive some education in hospital but I believed that what Mark needed was a place at a school for the severely handicapped. Quite how I set about this I can not now remember but after considerable enquiries I came to the conclusion that The Lord Mayor Treloar School near Basingstoke looked like the prefect solution. Dr. Tom Denning, the registrar to the Professor of Psychiatry, who had been assigned to help with some of my disturbed patients, agreed to take Mark to the school for a visit and assess if it was indeed suitable and to ascertain if they could cope with Mark's problems. The visit was a success and I applied to Mark's educational authority asking them to send him to this school. This was considered to be too expensive an option and the request was turned down. Most authorities, with a budget to consider, will always choose the most economical option but the one thing of which they are afraid is unfavourable publicity by the media. I therefore suggested to Mark that, with his typing machine, which he managed with one finger, he should write to Esther Rantzen, who at that time was interested in a small boy with liver problems in Addenbrooke's Hospital, explaining to her his situation. This he did. I tidied up his tape, glued it to a card and posted it off. Now I fear I must rely on speculation as Mark did not get an answer himself but, shortly afterwards the relevant Education Authority wrote to say that Mark could go to the Lord Mayor School. This proved to be a success and he stayed there till he was eighteen years old, after which his local authority settled him in a flat for the disabled with a befriender to help him and this arrangement has worked well ever since. Both Mark and myself are most grateful for this and, I suspect, we also owe thanks to Esther Rrantzen for a timely intervention.

A few days before I was due to retire, while I was discussing a problem with a colleague from the hospital biochemical laboratory, I was interrupted by the newly elected Regius Professor of Physic who, together with his entourage, thrust himself into my laboratory and announced, *'I am Professor Peters, I have come to see how much space I get when you retire'* I thought this was somewhat discourteous. My final day at work came on 30th September 1987, I found it a traumatic experience, I discharged my last patient on that day and handed over all my patients notes to the Records Officer who wheeled a trolley load a way with a glint of satisfaction at recovering what she considered to be her lost charges. Previously I had kept them all in my office to ensure that they were always readily available and did not disappear into some bottomless pit which seems to be present in most records department, from whence they would eventually reappear in some disorder. Often in University departments senior members, on retirement, if they have achieved distinction in their particular field, are offered some continuing facilities, but my search for such an arrangement was not productive. However, almost at the last minute Dr. Elsie Widdowson, the surviving half of the famous McCance-Widdson combination, who had a large room at the end of the University corridor offered me half of her room into which I could move all my own books and records and I certainly owe her thanks for this. This gave me a few months to wind down. There were other sweeping changes at this time as new Regius Professor of Physic was due to take office and the Professor of Medicine was due to retire the year after me. My tenure in Elsie Widdowson's room was therefore limited until we were both expelled to make way for other talent. It was unfortunate that I had signally failed to find a satisfactory solution as to whom to hand over my patients though two, who lived locally, continued to be cared for at Addenbrookes Hospital. Jill, unfortunately, with disastrous results as she subsequently suffered a recurrence of trientine induced renal damage. The physician who took over her care ignored my advice to make a regular check of her renal function and allowed her to suffer further severe renal damage. She gained a lot of weight from fluid retention but this was attributed to over eating and Jill was told to loose weight, a serious medical misdiagnosis. She finally escaped to my clinic in London where I reestablished molybdate treatment but unfortunately her kidney function was too damaged to recover spontaneously. After this she moved, with her husband, to Bristol but died of kidney failure whilst awaiting a suitable kidney for transplantation. A very sad ending to a long saga very bravely born.

In the summer of 1988, though it was entirely unplanned and, I may say, entirely unexpected, a solution to the future care of my little flock was forthcoming, which, after some careful thought, I readily grabbed with both hands, but this I will describe later.

CHAPTER 7

Medicolegal Problems

As the doctors say of a wasting disease, to start with it is easy to cure but difficult to diagnose; after a time,
unless it has been diagnosed and treated at the outset, it becomes easy to diagnose but difficult to cure.
Niccolo Machiavelli, The Prince. Trans. George Bull.

Abstract: The average delay in making the correct diagnosis for all patients was 2 years; some were diagnosed relatively quickly others waited many years. This resulted in some unnecessary deaths and some patients being left with severe disabilities and wanting compensation. I was involved in six such cases. In four cases, with the help of my evidence substantial damages were obtained but in two cases, which I think resulted in miscarriages of justice, the patient failed to obtain damages. My first case was in 1974 when a father complained of the late diagnosis of his son's illness which resulted in the boy's death He wanted publicity more than damages in the hope that such an error would not recur. The case was settled out of court with no publicity. Success was also achieved for twins from Belfast and for a civil engineer from England whose diagnosis had been made in the USA having been missed by his consultant in this country. The case of one unfortunate patient who suffered from a very rare abnormality of copper metabolism actually was settled the High Court in the Strand with the award of over one million pounds damages. In two cases my evidence failed to obtain damages, one of these was of a very bad case of case of medical incompetence by a psychiatrist but the plaintiff made her claim too late and the case never came to court. I recommended, in vain, an ex gratia payment should be made.

When Machiavelli wrote those lines he might have been writing about patients with Wilson's disease. My experience, from patients referred to me, was that the average delay in making the correct diagnosis was approaching two years. This means that although some patients may have been diagnosed reasonably quickly in many cases it took a good deal longer. Inevitably this resulted in some unnecessary deaths or, in other cases, permanent disability' in consequence of this some patients sought compensation via the courts. As a result I was asked to write reports in support of their claims and, in one case give evidence in the High Court in the Strand. The first such occasion was in 1974 when I was asked to report on the case of a 12 year old boy who had recently died of liver failure. His illness had started about a year earlier when the local paediatrician had diagnosed him as suffering from juvenile cirrhosis of the liver. His condition continued to deteriorate slowly. Eventually, on father's insistence, he was referred to the regional teaching hospital where, eventually, a diagnosis of Wilson's disease was made, but by then it was too late and he died shortly afterwards. Father wanted to sue the local paediatrician for negligence, not so much, he told me, for financial recompense, but to make the case public so that such mistakes would not occur again; what a hope. The barrister he employed, who was also medically qualified, came up to Cambridge to discuss the case with me. What neither of us could understand was why only the first hospital was to be sued as the teaching hospital did not appear to have made the diagnosis as soon as they should. However the case was settled out of court with modest damages for the father. Unfortunately he did not achieve his objective of obtaining publicity as a result of the out of court settlement. But there was one great benefit for the family. I arranged to screen the two younger siblings. A nine year old daughter and her six year old brother. The brother proved to be normal but the sister had the typical biochemical findings of presymptomatic Wilson's disease. I immediately started her on treatment with penicillamine and her abnormal liver tests soon returned to normal. She has remained well ever since and qualified in medicine before emigrating to the United States, but we still keep in touch.

My next case involved a pair of identical twins from Northern Ireland. At the time I first saw them they were 21 years of age and physically so dissimilar that I sent blood samples both to the Medical Research Council's (MRC) Laboratory for Human Biochemical Genetics and to

John Walshe (Ed.)

their Blood Group Unit. Both laboratories found that the twins were indeed identical. Both certainly had the biochemical lesion for Wilson's disease though only one was clinically affected. Arthur, the affected twin, at this stage could not talk but brought a comprehensive history from his referring physician. His illness had started some five years earlier with abnormal movements. He was referred to a psychiatrist who treated him with antidepressants and electroconvulsive therapy at, according to mother, £150 a time. His illness progressed slowly until he became bedridden and helpless, unable to talk or to swallow. At this stage he was admitted to an intensive care unit under the care of a physician who immediately made the correct diagnosis. His twin brother remained clinically unaffected and, whilst in Cambridge, actually got a job as a bouncer in a night club!

For legal reasons this case needed the opinion of a psychiatrist as well as myself and together we flew to Belfast. But this was the time of the troubles and I had no ambition to subject myself to the risk of being blown up. We insisted that we met the legal team at the airport and had our discussions there. These were successfully concluded and as this was a clear case of medical negligence, I would say incompetence: it was settled out of court for a considerable sum of money which was richly deserved but as scant compensation for a ruined life.

The next patient involved with the law was a 32 year old man, a civil, engineer who suffered from tremor of the head and arms which severely handicapped his earning capacity. He had been treated for some years as a case of familial tremor by a consultant neurologist. On a visit to the United States he sought medical advice and was at once correctly diagnosed as Wilson's disease. With my help he also reached an out of court settlement though I thought the damages awarded were not in keeping with what he had suffered. At the time of the court case his London neurologist had died which probably added difficulties to a very problematical defence. Fortunately he made a good recovery once treatment was started.

Shortly after I started work at the Middlesex Hospital and in 1988 I became involved in a much more interesting case. It resulted from a serious diagnostic error and seriously misguided surgical intervention. Paul was a 42 year old man with a responsible job and a family to support. He developed a sleep disturbance and fell asleep at the wheel of his car resulting in a relatively minor accident. He was admitted to a neurosurgical unit where they found he had diabetes and some rather doubtful neurological signs. The report on his brain scan said that there was a lesion in the mid brain, possibly a tumor and some changes in the motor centres suggesting a metabolic disease, either Wilson's disease or haemachromatosis, that is an iron storage disease. Blood samples were sent to the laboratory to investigate the possibility of a metabolic disease, but with out waiting for the results a neurosurgeon instructed his registrar to perform a biopsy on the suspected mid brain tumor, Eleven needle punctures of this region gave no useful information but caused him to have a disastrous brain haemorrhage which left him permanently very seriously disabled. In lay terms he was turned into a cabbage.

When the results of the blood tests were received they gave equivocal answers as to the questions of both metabolic diseases under investigation; that is the levels of copper and copper carrying protein were very low and the level of the iron carrying protein was very high ! Did he indeed have both the metabolic diseases suggested by the brain scan? At that stage I was asked as to the possibility of Wilson's disease, to which I replied that the evidence was insufficient and that a liver biopsy was necessary. This advice was ignored and treatment for Wilson's disease was started ! After a year of futile treatment his condition inevitably remained unchanged. His wife then brought Paul to see me. As he had been on anticopper treatment for a year it was impossible to interpret his results, though I was able to confirm that his serum copper and copper-protein were indeed very low. However there was virtually no copper in his urine. I therefore stopped his treatment for Wilson's disease and said I would repeat the tests in a year's time. As I predicted this year with no treatment did not result in the signs of Wilson's disease appearing but the tests, when repeated were unchanged. A liver biopsy showed that his liver copper was not raised, as in Wilson's disease but was actually lower than normal. At this stage legal proceedings were started. I thought the case was indefensible but the neurosurgeon in charge refused to admit any fault so the case actually came to court. I appeared as a witness in the High Court in the Strand. I only attended the one day so I did not hear the judge's summing up. My impression in court was that the Counsel for the defence did no really understand the situation and asked me a lot of irrelevant questions until the judge intervened. The outcome was that Paul won his case and was awarded very heavy damages. Interestingly enough the story did not end there. About a year later an article appeared in a medical journal describing a pair of brothers with a hitherto undescribed disease with diabetes and, in the late 40s changes in behaviour and tremor. The biochemical basis was an absence of the copper carrying protein caeruloplasmin and an associated overload of iron in the liver and a raised iron protein (ferretin) in the blood. This new disease was named 'acaeruloplasminaemia'. Paul had these findings and a liver scan confirmed the presence an excess of iron. It was thus possible to make a confident diagnosis that he did indeed suffer from this 'new' very rare metabolic disease. As there was no known treatment this hardly helped; I thought that perhaps regular infusions of caeruloplasmin should be given, but this presented many problems and as it could not hope to reverse the effects of his surgically induced brain haemorrhage the idea was not pursued further.

Thus, at that time I had been successful in getting damages for all the patients I had supported. However my next case was a failure. Very briefly it was of a boy whose Wilson's disease had been diagnosed rather late. His initial response to treatment was of an increase in symptoms but after a couple of months he showed real signs of improvement. Unfortunately, at this juncture his doctors, and there were far too many looking after him, doubled his dose of penicillamine. God only knows why they did this, and the deterioration seen initially returned. From then on things went from bad to worse. The defence was that some patients do badly what ever treatment they are given and he was one such. He may well have been one such, there is no means of knowing what would have happened if he had been properly treated. I felt that the crucial mistake was doubling his dose of penicillamine and then not trying alternative treatment with trientine until it was too late. The case never came to court, in a preliminary review of the evidence the judge found for the defence. I felt the benefit of the doubt should have gone to the patient and this was probably a miscarriage of justice.

The next case I wish to discuss demonstrates the speed, or lack there of, at which the law works. It also illustrates yet another case of a miscarriage of justice and how easily this can occur. The story begins with a 12 year old girl who developed a severe anaemia and mild jaundice. Her general practitioner referred her to a chest physician, an unusual decision, who diagnosed infective hepatitis without doing the necessary tests to confirm the diagnosis. The information about this stage of her illness is, to say the least sketchy. All her case notes had been destroyed and only a few doctors letters remained to try and assess what actually happened. At some stage soon after this she was referred to a general surgeon who noted that she was improving and no further action was required. Five years later she developed a speech defect, problems with writing and unsteadiness in walking shortly after being involved in a road traffic accident. She was referred to a neurologist who made a diagnosis of hysteria following her involvement in the car accident. She was then referred to a psychiatrist in a geriatric hospital ! where the diagnosis of hysteria was confirmed. She saw at least two different psychiatrists who were happy with the diagnosis and she was admitted to a psychiatric hospital for treatment. It was noted that she had episodes of temper and a difficult relationship with her parents After a while she realised that the treatment she was receiving was doing her no good and, in my view very wisely, she discharged herself.

The patient then left home and went to live with an aunt in a city some distance away where there was a teaching hospital. She took with her a referral to the consultant psychiatrist. He admitted her to his hospital and without questioning he accepted the diagnosis of hysteria and continued to treat her accordingly. Meanwhile her neurological symptoms progressed to leave her severely disabled physically. She also had, by now, serious personality difficulties leading to friction with her contemporaries and life style was disintegrating. A year later a new registrar was appointed to the psychiatric unit who immediately made the correct diagnosis of Wilson's disease.

I was asked by the legal representatives of the Regional Health Authority to defend the case. Having reviewed her by now very extensive case notes, some 1,200 pages in all, I gave them my opinion that this was one of the worst cases of medical negligence I had ever met with and that they should settle out of court in order to avoid wasting money on a long drawn out and futile defence from which only the lawyers would benefit.

Four years later I was informed by the solicitors that the case had been struck out of court because there was too long a delay in making a claim. I wrote back saying '*To be quite honest I was shocked by the mismanagement of this case. The patient would now seem to have been deprived of a normal youth by her doctors and now she is to be denied compensation by the law. In my view this is an effrontery to natural justice and I can only recommend that the Health Authority makes this patient a generous ex gratia payment'* I heard no more. I have very little doubt that my advice was not taken. A lawyer once said to me '*You do not go to court for justice, you go for a settlement'.* How true.

It is clearly apparent from this last case just how long the law can take before reaching a decision however satisfactory or unsatisfactory this may be. In 2002 that distinguished jurist, Dame Elizabeth Butler-Sloss, in an address to The Royal Society of Medicine, blamed medical expert witnesses for all the delays in settling medico-legal disputes. This has not been my experience. In all the cases in which I have been involved there seems to have been no sense of urgency in the legal profession that a seriously disabled claimant needs compensation for an act of medical negligence. It must be admitted that to prepare a report in such a case may require sorting through more than a thousand pages of photocopied, scarcely legible hospital notes. These can comprise doctors scrawl, equally illegible nurses reports, also reports from physiotherapists, occupational therapists and social workers. In addition there are laboratory reports, radiological reports, temperature charts and drug charts together with doctors letters, all put together in no more than a semblance of chronological order. Thus a report can not be produced quickly, but if Dame Butler-Sloss really believes that delays are all due to the medical profession she lives in a parallel universe. Not only are lawyers at least equally guilty of causing delay but also, in my experience, they show no great enthusiasm in paying for the work involved.

The last case with which I was involved was quite different. I was approached by American firm of Attorneys for help in the case of a Peruvian peasant ! The story was that this unfortunate young man was sleeping by the roadside in his village in the Andes when a truck from a US based mining firm shed large amounts of mercury. Shortly afterwards he developed a rash and pain in his hands and fingers and later tremor. He reported sick and was given two injections of 'Neurobion', whatever that is. The tremor increased and he and other villagers, presumably with similar symptoms, were diagnosed as suffering from mercury poisoning, as they probably were at that time, and were treated with penicillamine. This he received for the following eight months. This was a strange choice of treatment, probably based on minimum cost to the firm, and certainly not the drug of first choice for mercury poisoning. His condition continued to deteriorate and he was finally admitted to a hospital in Lima completely helpless and bedridden. Some four years later he was seen by two visiting physicians from the United States who made a firm diagnosis of Wilson's disease.

In my report I concluded that exposure to mercury hastened the onset of symptoms of Wilson's disease, two heavy metals being more damaging to the brain than one alone. That penicillamine was not the drug of choice for treatment of mercury poisoning and that the correct diagnosis was disastrously delayed by the episode of mercury intoxication. The case was eventually settled in favour of the patient. I found the United States Attorneys much more business-like and much easier to cooperate with than their English counter parts.

CHAPTER 8

The End of a Strained Relationship

And short retirement urges sweet return.
Milton, Paradise Lost.

Abstract: September in the year 1987 heralded my retirement both as a reader in the University and also that of my honorary appointment as a consultant physician to Addenbrooke's Hospital. At that time I had been unable to make any satisfactory arrangements for the continued specialist care of my patients. A solution was offered in the following summer when Dr Gerald Stern invited me to set up a Wilson's disease clinic at University College Hospital (UCH) in London. One problem had to be solved as to who would do the specialist studies of copper metabolism The UCH laboratory was not able to undertake the preferred method of caeruloplasmin estimation but Scheinberg agreed to do this for me if I mailed him suitable samples to New York. My clinic ran in conjunction with Dr Stern's out patient clinic until we transferred to the Middlesex Hospital and Dr Lees took over from Dr Stern on his retirement. My expenses for the travel to London were met by Aldrich Chemicals, who had taken over the production of Trientine. There were problems over the account of an overseas patient and also a major problem when two Cambridge doctors published results culled from my case notes.. Eventually I tendered my resignation on reaching the age of 80 years and handed over the clinic to Dr. Godfrey Gillett who had joined me some years before. There is also an account of my somewhat unhappy relationship with the University of Cambridge

Unlike so many doctors, disillusioned by the stultifying bureaucracy of the NHS, the countless unrealistic targets and the hostile attitude of the Government to the profession. who now eagerly await retirement, I hated giving up the care of my patients and the research involved. I felt I had lost my purpose in life. It was with great regret that I discharged my last patient and moved out of my laboratory cum office. There was decorating to be done about the home and a large garden to look after but these activities were not intellectually satisfying and I worried about the essentially non-specialist care my patients would inevitably receive from the various doctors who would now look after them and who could not be expected to know the minutiae of Wilson disease and its management. By the summer of 1988 I had redecorated the spare bedroom and bathroom and also the dining room and the garden was under control There was some unreported work to be written up and published after which I wondered how I would fill my time usefully. Then, to my surprise and delight, I was contacted by Dr, Gerald Stern, consultant neurologist at my old stamping ground, University College Hospital. He was visiting Cambridge as an examiner for the final medical qualifying examination and he had a proposal which might enable me to continue my work. We met for a snack lunch in the University Combination Room, a common room for fellows, where he said he thought it a great pity that my particular talent should be wasted and would I like to start a clinic for Wilson disease patients at his hospital? He had funds from a private endowment which would meet my expenses for doing this. He would need to clear this with the hospital board and, if this proved acceptable, I could join his weekly out patients clinic and if any Wilson's disease patients required admission they could be accommodated in his beds or in the metabolic ward where I had worked, with Boris Senior, on cystinuria some 40 years earlier,. From my point of view the question was this, could a sufficient number of my former patients be persuaded to come to London to make the enterprise worth while. I decided to give it a go. Meanwhile the hospital authorities were not too keen on the project: they were worried about the effect setting up of a new clinic might have on their budget! They did not seem to realize that they might actually make money by charging the overseas patients who could be expected to attended my clinic This problem was overcome by Dr Stern arranging for me to have an honorary senior lectureship at near by University College, London, situated conveniently just across the road in Gower Street. As a result of these negotiations the new clinic started later the same year.

Another problem that had to be solved was who would carry out the specialist biochemical estimations for copper in body fluids and, more difficult, that of the copper carrying serum protein, caeruloplasmin, deficient in all Wilson disease patients. I offered to do these myself if laboratory space could be found, but this suggestion came to naught. Fortunately the Professor of Clinical Biochemistry in charge of the hospital laboratory was my old friend, Freddie Flynn who would be responsible for most of the routine tests and he assigned one of his chemists to undertake the copper protein determinations; although I was not entirely happy about the method to be employed, it tended to give false high results, it was better than nothing. The sophisticated method I had employed was simply not suitable for a routine laboratory to set up for a very small number of patients. The copper determinations, for blood and urine, would be made by the biochemist in the metabolic ward. Additional help came when Herb Scheinberg who, with extraordinary generosity, offered to do the blood copper and caeruloplasmin estimations for me, with out charge, if I mailed him serum at the end of each clinic. Thus I obtained all these results in duplicate. This compromise worked out very well and lasted till both he and I finally retired in the year 2000; furthermore this duplication caused no friction with my new colleagues in London.

I wrote round to my former patients and before long the clinic was booked up for several weeks in advance. I caught an early 125 intercity train from Huntingdon to Kings Cross, only a 35 minutes journey, whence a short ride on the underground to Euston Square station got me to UCH in plenty of time for the morning clinic. This was a relatively relaxed affair with a stop mid morning for coffee when we all joined up in Gerald Stern's room to discuss problems. It was interesting to renew my connection with the metabolic ward where I had worked with Boris Senior in the early 1950s. Here by hangs a tale. This ward built just 100 years ago, had originally been a children's ward with coloured tiles around the walls showing pictures of nursery rhymes. After its conversion to a metabolic ward and laboratories it was found that radioisotope studies were made difficult by the very high background counts. When this was investigated it was found that the yellow pigment in the coloured tiles was uranium based ! Most unsuitable for children, clearly not understood at the time of construction. At the end of the morning I would leave all the blood specimens I had collected in the hospital laboratory, get a quick bite in University College common room and return to the hospital to deal with the clinic letters, retrieve my share of the serum from the laboratory and package this up for posting on to Dr Scheinberg, then catch the 125 train back home. After about a year this particular service was discontinued and I was reduced to using a standard commuter cattle train. I was ever intrigued at Kings Cross to see that the station clock was always a few minutes ahead of that at the neighbouring, and much lauded, St Pancras station. I liked to think that the explanation was that Rail Track based its time on the sun and not Greenwich, hence the difference in time as St Pancras was about 100 yards west of Kings Cross and there fore gave a slightly earlier time, more likely explanation was that one of the clocks was wrong. On approaching Kings Cross I remembered Chesterton's delightful poem about the station ending with that evocative last line '***What poet race shot such cyclopean arches to the stars'.***

Many of the more complex procedures I had previously carried out had to be abandoned but it was possible to gather sufficient data to give top class clinical care, though research was ruled out. After a couple of years Gerald Stern told me that his ability to fund my expenses from his private endowment was over but I was able to replace this by approaching the makers of trientine who kindly agreed to continue covering my travel expenses.

The next upheaval came when UCH was closed down or, to be more accurate, was turned into a research centre in cooperation with University College and we all moved to the near by Middlesex Hospital; at about the same time Gerald Stern retired and his place was taken over by Andrew Lees, who was later appointed Professor of Neurology. This made little difference to me personally except that my journey from King's Cross to the Middlesex Hospital added one further stop to my underground journey, that is to Great Portland Street, and the further walk to the hospital was somewhat longer than that from Euston Square to University College Hospital.

In 1989 I found myself, unexpectedly, involved in a distinctly unpleasant incident. As I have said, when I left Addenbrooke's Hospital I returned all my case notes, with the results of all relevant research data, to the hospital records department. I later discovered that two of my former colleagues on the hospital staff had taken these case notes and proposed to published a long article on Wilson disease, largely based on my work, in a medical journal, The Acta Neurologica Scandinavica in which they referred to '…our own 195 cases.'. They also used all my research data as if it was their own. I had reason to suspect that this was going on and had written to the senior author forbidding him to publish my results, a letter which he ignored. When the article was published Dr Scheinberg was so incensed that he wrote to the editor of the journal in question and his letter was published in full which I here quote. This appeared in print in volume 81 of The Acta in 1990.

Readers of Acta Neurologica Scandinavica should be aware of certain facts relating to the article 'Wilson;s disease; clinical groups in 400 cases' by TR Denning and GE Berrios (1989; 80: 527-534). Of the 400 cases 205 were from published series of none of which was either Denning or Berrios the author. They refer to the remaining patients as 'our own' In truth, however, all 195 were cases of John Walshe who had, in writing, prohibited these authors from utilizing his clinical records for this article.

Over the past 35 years I have cooperated closely with Walshe in the investigation of Wilson's disease. He is, and has long been, the world's leading expert on the treatment of that rare inherited disease. He discovered the only two drugs, penicillamine and triethylene tetramine dihydrochloride, that are approved by the U.S. Food and Drugs Administration as safe and effective therapy for Wilson's disease. These drugs have converted this inherited disorder from one whose outcome is always an early death into one in which patients, if diagnosed in early childhood, can virtually be assured of life of normal length and health.

As a direct result of these therapeutic triumphs, as well as of the important advances he has made in our understanding of the natural history and pathogenesis of Wilson's disease, Walshe has created a unique data base from the very large number of patients with this disease who came to his clinic in Cambridge from all over the world. The 195 cases, which Denning and Berrios have arrogated, constitute the essence of Walshe's life work and his significant contribution to knowledge.

The unauthorised utilization and publication of a scientist's data constitute perhaps the most serious breach of the code of conduct that should exist between scientists.
 I.H. Scheinberg

When Scheinberg wrote to the Vice Chancellor of the University pointing out these facts the reply he received was that '**No inappropriate behaviour had occurred'**. It seemed to me that this was just another example of the Establishment white washing itself, and here the matter died. To be honest I was disappointed but life must go on and this, apart from its effect upon my blood pressure, really made no difference to my situation.

I had always found that it was important to establish the best possible relations with the service departments, laboratories, radiology, physiotherapy and others. It was my custom to visit them in person, describe the reasons for my requests if these were in any way unusual and also discussed the results. This had worked well at Addenbrooke's, at UCH and now at the Middlesex. This reminds me of an incident at Addenbrookes when I queried some results with the principal biochemist. *Why, he asked, are you the only physician who ever does this*. The only reply I could think of was '*Perhaps I am the only physician who studies your reports*' I suspect there may well have been a basis of truth in this suggestion. Another incident, at the Middlesex Hospital, occurred shortly after they had installed a new top of the range MRI scanner. I had gone down to discuss the findings with the radiologist in charge when I found two of my former Addenbrookes colleagues in the Department studying the new machine. I took the opportunity to quip '*Hello, have you come down from the provinces to see how things are done properly at a top London Hospital*'.

I have little doubt that my new clinic, which had now become firmly established in London, was a success; not only had most of my old patients been pleased to sign up but the flow of new patients was soon re-established both from at home and abroad. The overseas patients engendered an unexpected set of difficulties. They were not entitled to free hospital care under the Health Service unless that brought the Common Market form e114 and I always took pains to explain to them, before they came, that they should arm themselves with one of these forms if possible, if not they would be subject to certain basic charges over which I had no control, these covered attendance at the clinic and certain basic laboratory determinations, all other investigations were charged in addition. I recommended that as many of these tests as possible, should be done at the referring hospital and that they should bring the results with them. I also informed the clerk in charge of out patient bookings when an overseas patient was due. Unfortunately these charges were not always collected, for which I was sometimes blamed. However I felt I was not the hospital's debt collector and that, having given prior notice, I had no further responsibility.

On one occasion this led to a major row nearly leading to my suspension. The patient in question was the daughter of a citizen from one of the Arab Sheikdoms whose elder sister had recently died of Wilson disease. After diagnosis the sister had been treated with penicillamine and also, for an intercurrent infection, with penicillin. The combination of these two drugs had led to suppression of her bone marrow and she died of fulminant infection. Father and a companion, plus daughter, heavily veiled, arrived in my clinic with evidence from the referring physician that strongly supported the diagnosis that she also had Wilson disease, in the presymptomatic stage. After taking the history through the companion who acted as an interpreter, I requested to examine the patient's abdomen. After a long discussion between father and interpreter I was gravely informed that, under the circumstances, this was permissible. Having assessed the various therapeutic options I decided that the only therapy likely to be available in their home country was penicillamine. I therefore had little option, I need to treat the girl with this drug despite the fact that it had probably contributed, in some way, to her sisters death. To avoid unnecessary risk I arranged for her to have twice weekly blood counts to cover the first few weeks of treatment. I discussed this with the house physician who was to undertake this task. He was to inform me at once if these tests showed any evidence of bone marrow damage. Unfortunately this young doctor was over enthusiastic and, in addition to the routine blood counts, he ordered a repetition of all the tests I carried out on a first visit which, under the circumstance, were quite uncalled for. Thus, by the end of a couple of weeks father was confronted with a huge bill which he could not possibly pay and in fact he made no attempt to do so. The biochemist now in charge, my friend Freddie Flynn having retired, was not prepared to let his payment lapse. I went up to his room to discuss the problem and was saddened to find he was more interested in his budget than the welfare of a patient. The matter was eventually resolved in favour of the patient as it was realized that the tests had not been officially sanctioned and were not germane to the patients management. However the episode caused a lot of ill feeling and I suspect resulted in the administration putting a black mark against my name. Being only an honorary physician and a guest at the hospital I was not in a strong position to say what I felt about the whole episode, but in the long run it appeared to be forgotten. I suspect I owe a lot to Gerald Stern's diplomacy for the solution of this clash with the system.

The year 1994 proved to be very rewarding. A quite unexpected honour was forthcoming, I as awarded the honorary degree of MD by the University of Uppsala. I had connections with the University Hospital in that city having lectured there some years earlier and corresponded with Dr. Kerstin Westermark, their Wilson disease expert. Uppsala is an ancient University (Fig. **11**) situated somewhat north of Stockholm. It has a river running through the centre of the town and a fine cathedral in which is to be found the tomb of the warrior king, Gustavus Adolphus. The degree giving ceremony was impressive and each degree was signaled by the firing of a canon outside the hall. I have subsequently treasured the gold ring that came with the degree, but the top hat I have found no further occasion to wear. It all made up for the MD degree the University of Cambridge and denied me 40 years earlier.

Another salutary story is worth mentioning here. It is of a school girl who suffered deteriorating performance at school, a change in her voice and the development of movement disorders. After a difficult eighteen months Wilson's disease was diagnosed and she was referred to a specialist neurological hospital where she was started on penicillamine. A week later she developed a rash and fever. The drug was stopped and later reintroduced in a smaller dose, but with out either steroid or antihistamine cover. Inevitably the rash recurred. The drug was again stopped and trientine substituted. On this she started to improve slowly but her doctors wished to hasten recovery and added zinc sulphate to her regime. This had two unfortunate side effects. First the trientine combined with the zinc, reducing the efficacy of both and second it resulted in the development of a very severe anaemia which was missed. As a result the patient deteriorated rapidly to a condition of near helplessness very similar to that of the Greek patient previously described.. Her mother realized the seriousness of the situation and brought Lisa to my clinic. I realized, at once, that drastic action needed to be taken and her treatment completely revised. This put me in a very difficult position; I could not appropriate a patient not officially referred and to have done so to a very distinguished professor would have been tantamount to professional suicide. However a rather unusual solution to the problem was at hand. Her father was a banker, at that time working in New York. I therefore said to mother. get tickets on the next flight to New York and go and see Dr. Scheinberg at the Albert Einstein Hospital. I will ring him up and explain what is happening and telling him of the severe anaemia which has precipitated the problem. If any one can help Lisa, he can. Mother took my advice and made the journey early the following week. Lisa was treated in New York with penicillamine, reintroduced under steroid cover, and a course of BAL. She made an excellent recovery and eventually returned to my clinic. My involvement in this somewhat unprofessional activity has hitherto been kept a dark secret.

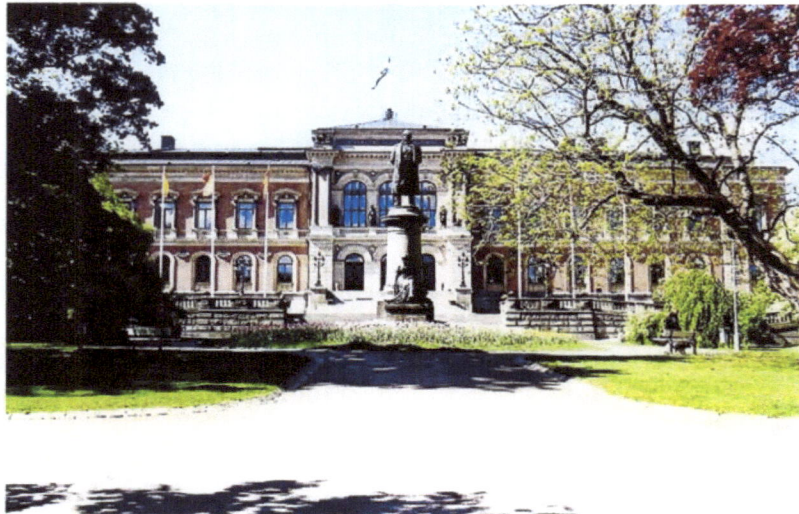

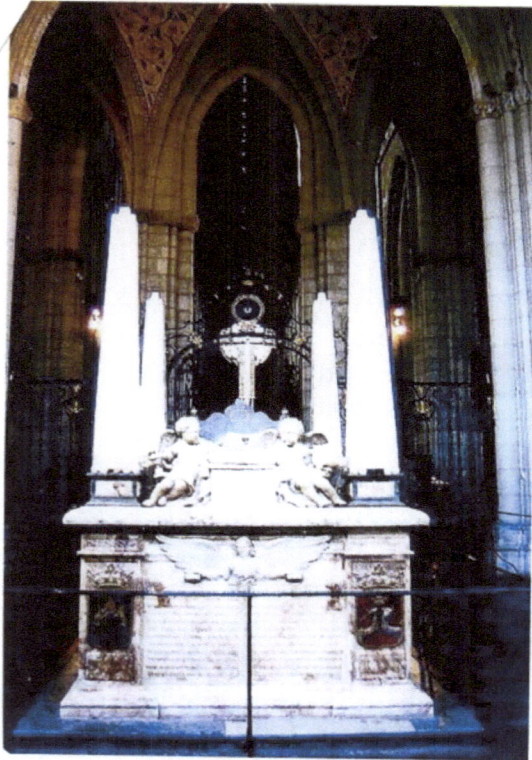

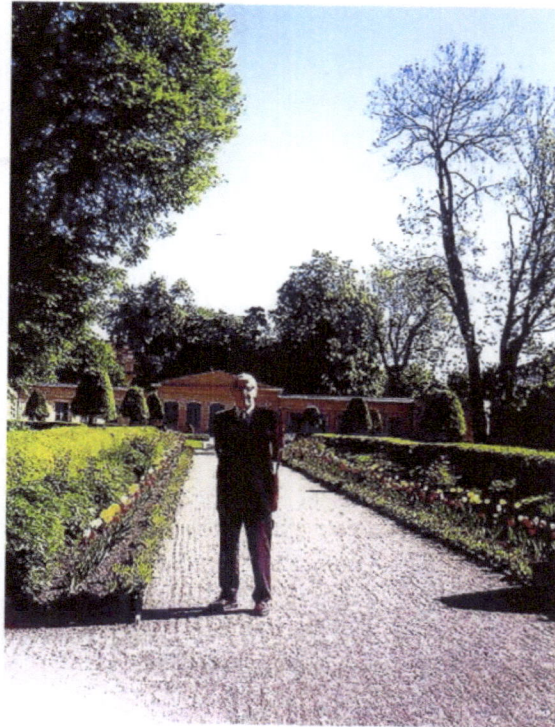

Fig. (11). Uppsala.

(1)   The University building where the Degree ceremony was held
(2)   The Tomb of Gustavus Adolphus in the Cathedral
(3)   Myself in Linnaeus' Garden

Apart from moving into a brand new out patient clinic things went smoothly for the following years. However the ever creeping bureaucracy of the health Service, from time to time, intruded. The one which particularly irritated me was the 'pink form' This had to be filled in for every out patient, the time of arrival, the time of the appointment, the time they were seen, the time of departure, tests ordered, etc. No patient was to wait for more than half an hour, thus breaching the Government's target, otherwise an official rebuke was to be expected. Some parts of the form should have been filled in by the clerks, such as name age address and hospital number and time of arrival. They never were. As I never found it possible to keep to a tight time schedule most patients breached the half hour wait of the government target. It was my policy to allow every patient as much time as I needed and they wanted for a consultation. After all most had come considerable distances and did not wish to be put through a sausage machine. I always apologized for delays and explained my reason. I really believe that my patients preferred this to a brief official time slot. I never had any complaints. Hence I kept all the pink forms till the end of the clinic and then filled them up to a theoretical schedule so that no patient appeared to have waited more than 29 minutes! No doubt the pink forms went to some office in hospital management, were correlated and sent on the Ministry and all concerned glowed with pride at this wonderful system that had banished waiting times and was working so well. I have no means of knowing how my colleagues treated these forms, they may have been more compliant. I was always something of a rebel against the establishment.

Unquestionably the best thing that happened in this period was that I was joined in my clinic by Dr Godfrey Gillett. At that time he was a medical registrar at The Hospital for Sick Children, Great Ormond Street where he was a clinical biochemist with a particular interest in inherited metabolic disease. He had been coming to the Middlesex Hospital to sit in on Dr Brinton's clinic for patients with metabolic bone disease when he decided to learn about Wilson disease. This proved to be a very happy move. Godfrey quickly learned how I ran the clinic and also proved to be a very helpful associate and his presence kept me up to date with developments in other fields of medicine with which I had lost touch. As the millennium approached I realized that the time was coming for me to retire. I was, at that stage, probably the last hospital doctor in practice who had been working since before the inauguration of the National Health Service in 1948, indeed the last of the dinosaurs ! I would be eighty in that year and I felt it would be better to retire gracefully rather than leave someone the invidious task of asking me to go, embarrassing for him and humiliating for me. I therefore tendered my resignation and suggested that Godfrey, who had by now come to know most of my patients and how I liked to investigate them and to monitored their progress, should take over the clinic. By this time he had himself achieved a consultant appointment at the Northern General Hospital in Sheffield and was well qualified to do this. He had, in fact, for some time, been coming down by train from Sheffield to London specially to sit in on my clinic. To my great pleasure this arrangement was accepted in a somewhat ad hoc fashion and has worked very successfully ever since. He now sees patients from the south of England at the newly constructed University College Hospital in London and those from the north at his hospital in Sheffield. Another successful development at this time was the formation of a support group, The Wilson's Disease Support Group UK (WDSG, UK) which is now run by two of my expatients and the group meets for an annual get together and circulates a twice yearly news letter, has a web site and can give advice and help to patients who may seem fit to make enquiries both from this country and from abroad. The final episode of my carreer proved to be a Festschrift, organized by Professor Andrew Lees, at the National Hospital Queen Square which was attended by many of my colleagues and co-workers in the Wilson disease field from Europe. This was followed by a splendid 80th Birthday party, organized by Ann, my wife, at which many of the festschrift delegates came to celebrate with me. It was a indeed fitting end to an unusually long and I would like to believe successful career.

Bemjamin Disraeli stated, in the House of Commons in 1873, '*A University should be a place of light, of liberty and of learning*'. And yet my relationship with this august body was not always of the happiest as must already have become apparent from earlier sections of this work. The University of Cambridge was my employer for some 30 years. There were several reasons for this lack of harmony. After some thought, I have decided to give an account of these differences. This strained relationship, I would like to think, did not affect the quality of my work, the results of which speak for themselves, nor my enthusiasm for it. I enjoyed a great deal of independence to channel my energies between research and patient care and what more can man want than to enjoy the work for which he is paid. There can be few in such a fortunate position and I am certainly grateful for this. Can it be only in a University setting that such be possible? Certainly I can not see the NHS permitting it: such a specialized effort would not be considered as cost effective in the eyes of either a chief administrator or his accountant.

My association with the University began as long ago as 1938 when, as still a school boy, I went up to Cambridge to sit the First MB examination. Having achieved this first step on the long road to a medical qualification I was accepted by Trinity Hall to start as a preclinical medical student in October 1939. However war was declared in September of that year and the University panicked and called all its first year medical students to start work immediately. How this was to help the war effort it is difficult to know, it certainly did not result in my qualifying a day earlier. Together with a small number of other young hopefuls I duly presented myself for this new venture. My most cherished memory of the following years was that I learned the then little known and arcane art of brass rubbing from Donald Missen who was in charge of the University collection kept in the Sedgwick Museum on the Downing Street site. Each week end, weather permitting, I would load my bicycle and set forth, with a roll of detail paper slung under the saddle and handle bars somewhat like a small torpedo and, armed with rubbing wax and a special graphite mixture, a secret of Donald Missen, to outline the stone in which the brass was set also delineate the outline of missing parts, the indent. One venture was to make a record of all the indents of lost brasses in Ely Cathedral some of which must have been quite splendid, particularly that of Alan of Walsingham, architect of the octagon. Very many years later I realized that the feet of the ever increasing number of those who now visit the cathedral were eroding these indents so that, as a record of what had been lost, they would soon cease to be of value. I therefore gave the entire collection to the Dean who, I believe, handed them on to the University library. I had expected them to be kept in the cathedral archives. But at least the record is now safe for posterity should any future researcher into the cathedral's history be interested. During my time in Cambridge I must have rubbed all the brasses within cycling distance of the city and a few more distant ones reached by local train. Another less happy memory is of the cold in my digs with ice on the inside of the windows during that first year of the war. The most important legacy of my time as an undergraduate was of my final year as a part II physiology student when I discovered the excitement of research from that great physiologist, Wilhelm Feldberg, one of a number of distinguished scientist who had escaped Hitler and found refuge in English universities. I suspect, though I did not realize, at the time, that this had a great deal to do with my subsequent career. I have been asked why I have not described any student binges, wartime students did not participate in such activities. Having passed the second MB examination I proceeded to the study of clinical medicines, as all Cambridge student had to do in those days, at a teaching hospital, in my case University College Hospital (UCH) in London where my father was consultant neurologist. My most vivid memory as a student relates to an incident when I was learning midwifery. I was assigned to a delivery on the district, that was Camden Town. It was late in 1944 when London was under attack from flying bombs and rockets. Deliveries on the district, as a consequence, were few and far between and this was a rare and valuable experience. As this particular labour progressed I could hear the drone of a flying bomb getting nearer and nearer, in fact frighteningly near, and then, the warning sign, the throb of the engine cut out. The instinct to get under the mother's bed was enormous but had to be resisted. Fortunately for us this particular bomb was destined for another target and, following the explosion, the delivery proceeded without further mishap. It was an interesting experience !

The next visits I needed to make to Cambridge were in December 1944 and June 1945 to take the two parts of the final MB examination which would qualify me to practice medicine. I still vividly recollect standing, with a large crowd of other hopefuls, on the staircase of the pathology department whilst Professor Dean, the professor of pathology, known to all as 'Daddy Dean', read out the list of successful candidates in alphabetical order and of getting more and more apprehensive as he slowly worked his way down the alphabet to the Ws. The relief in hearing my name read out was immense. We were not, as I had expected, asked to take the Hiporatic oath. In the train back to London I asked myself '*What have you let yourself in for now ? What adventures lie in wait and can you cope*?' A few days later I took up my first appointment as house physician to Professor Harold Himsworth. This lasted six months and earned my first pay cheque, £120 for six months work with out a single official day off, but I enjoyed every minute of it. It was in this six months, with much more responsibility than is allowed to junior these days, that I really learned medicine the hard way. I hope and trust this was not at the expense of those patients who came under my care at that time.

Although the long years of war ended in 1945, military service still lay in wait. My two years, as I have already mentioned, were spent in the Middle East and I acquired a lasting love of Greece and an interest in its history and monuments. One episode remains vividly in my memory. I received a temporary posting to a unit giving instruction to the reconstituted Greek army. We were based on the Gulf of Marathon. I suppose my role was to give assistance if any untrained solider managed to get himself shot. During the exercises I would sit in my ambulance with the Greek interpreter. He was, I believe, a Professor from the University of Athens. I happened to be reading the Iliad at the time, a copy of which I had picked up in a bookshop in Athens. He asked if I could check his English pronunciations if he read from this to me. All went well but one evening he was heard to remark to the Commanding Officer '*Your young officers are mostly silly boys, but your doctor, he is an intellectual*': I wish I had this in writing ! I also managed to break my big toe on a hidden stone running into the gulf for a swim where my watch, not waterproof, perished as had the Persian army some 2,500 years earlier.

After demobilization I was able to rejoin the Medical Unit at UCH and the start, in a modest way in my research activities. By the year 1951 I had acquired enough data on the disturbances of aminoacid metabolism in patients with liver disease to write this work up for publication in that prestigious journal, The Quarterly Journal of Medicine (QJM). To my great satisfaction my manuscript was accepted with out modification. At this point Professor Rosenheim, the recently appointed head of the Unit, he had recently replaced professor Himsworth who had moved on to become Secretary of the Medical Research Council, advised me that I should submit my work as a thesis for the degree of MD at Cambridge. I suggested that as this was soon to appear as a publication it might make it ineligible as a thesis. A subject I referred to briefly earlier. Max assured that this would not matter as his own MD thesis had been based entirely on published work but it had been awarded the Raymond Horton Smith prize as the best thesis of the year.

Thus duly encouraged I decided to rewrite the results of my research in much greater detail and included all the experimental protocols. Having completed the work, I dispatched the completed thesis, in duplicate as required, to the office of the Regius Professor of Physic in Cambridge. At that time, in the early 1950s, the Regius was Sir Lionel Whitby who had risen to fame for doing Winston Churchill's blood count when he developed pneumonia in North Africa. At that time Sir Lionel was also Master of Downing College and Vice Chancellor of the University, a figure of great importance in university life. Soon after submitting my thesis, and by a most unfortunate coincidence, my paper appeared in print in the QJM. Shortly after this I received a letter with a Cambridge post mark which I eagerly opened expecting to find myself awarded an MD. After all Max had said that my thesis was, in his view, well above the average standard of those submitted. Imagine my shock and disappointment to read that the results of my labours was rejected on the ground that it consisted largely of published work. I showed this to Max who penned a letter for me to send to the Regius appealing against this decision. **'If you have any more trouble let me know and I will write to the Regius and sort things out'** he assured me. The Regius replied to my letter by inviting me to an interview in his rooms in The Master's Lodge in Downing College. I duly presented myself on time wondering what to expect but with little optimism as to the results. When I arrived Sir Lionel had, obviously from his dress, just returned from an official university function in the Senate House. He was with his secretary and duly kept me waiting long after the stated time until he had finished his dictating. I was then summoned into his inner sanctum with the unforgotten words, **'Come in young man, we are not pleased with you'**. This seemed me more the way to address an unruly undergraduate than a professional colleague. From then on things went from bad to worse. After some initial sparring I was told your thesis was rejected because **'You deliberately tried to deceive the examiners by submitting published work with out acknowledging it'. 'I beg your pardon',** I said, **'but unless there has been some terrible typing error you will find an acknowledgement on the front page, can you pass me the thesis so I can check on this'** He passed me the manuscript and I pointed out to him that there was indeed a due acknowledgement to the QJM on the front page. **'That'** he said **'does not count, all acknowledgements must be on the back page'** ! I was then told I must submit a new thesis and he would instruct me how to do so. That was more than I could take and I got up from my chair and said' **Thank you Sir Lionel but I have no intention of doing so. I have no reason to think that a second thesis would receive more fair treatment than the first and to rewrite the thesis would be entirely intellectual prostitution'** I left him speechless. Professor Dean, who had been master of my college, wrote to me to say that I had been rude to the Regius and I owed him an apology. I replied to the effect that the truth was seldom acceptable to those who are not accustomed to hear it and there I thought the matter would be laid to rest.

A year later, to my great surprise my new chief, Dr. John Stokes whose medical registrar I had recently become, returned from Cambridge where he had been an examiner in the final MB examination, He brought back, so he told me, a message for me from Sir Lionel Whitby. This was to the effect that the Regius thought the time had come for me to resubmit my work for the degree of MD. This seemed to me to be a bizarre state of affairs and I wrote to the Regius saying that I thought this was a most undignified way for him to do business and if he had anything to say to me he could do so in the usual way by letter. I had by now resigned any thought of achieving an MD and, having passed the examination of the Royal College of Physicians for membership of that august body felt I no longer needed the Cambridge degree. After these heated exchanges I must say it came as a considerable surprise when, in 1957, I was appointed to a post in the Department of Experimental Medicine at Cambridge, but by then Sir Lionel had died and been replaced by Professor Joseph Mitchell, the physician in charge of radiotherapy at Addenbrooke's Hospital. All was forgotten and forgiven, or was it?

Some years after I had become established in my new post and had risen from the lowly rank of Assistant Director of Research to that of Reader in Metabolic Disease I decided that I needed a doctorate to attain credibility in the University. It was alleged, at that time, that the most difficult doctorate to attain was that of Doctor of Science (ScD) awarded by the faculty of Biology B. I decided to have a go and submit reprints of all my published work, reprints of some 60 or 70 manuscripts in all. Before I took this step I consulted Sir Rudolph Peters who most kindly agreed to have a look at my dossier for me and having done so he encouraged me to proceed with the venture. At almost the same time, by another of those coincidences which seemed to dog my degree ambitions, Dr Leslie Cole who had been the assessor to the Regius and had signed the letter rejecting my original MD thesis, came up to me and asked why I did not submit my published work, now permissible under a new statue, for the degree of MD. I replied that having just submitted this for the degree of ScD I thought it would be most unwise to submit the same work for two degrees at the same time and risk being refused both on some other obscure statute that I was not aware of. My decision proved correct and I was duly awarded my ScD. It appeared that my caution was well justified. I no longer had need of an MD. But the drama did not end there. Later I was asked to assess an MD thesis, which presumably came within my corpus of expertise, submitted by some aspiring candidate. I declined to do so on the grounds that it would be quite inappropriate for an examiner, who had been refused that degree on the grounds that he had cheated, to act as an examiner for another candidate. I was told I was being childish but I feel sure that I was morally right to do so. Finally, as I have already described I was awarded an honorary MD by the University of Uppsala some forty years after the start of the drama, I felt at last that I had won the war as well as the argument.

When I took up my appointment with the University in October 1957 I hoped that I might be offered some association with my old college, Trinity Hall; dining rights in hall, perhaps. However there was a deathly silence. At the end of my first academic year, late in June 1958, I did receive a letter from the senior tutor of Trinity Hall saying that he had not been in touch before as he did not know how to do so. I, thought this quite an unlikely excuse. He invited me to dine with him in hall. Unfortunately the date he suggested was when I was to be on holiday in Florence, where Ann and I were to be the guests of one of my father's old patients. She lived in a beautiful 14th century palazzo overlooking Florence with a view to die for. I replied to the tutor thanking him for the invitation but explaining that I would be away at the time and perhaps something could be arranged for another date. I heard no more. Some 20 years later I received a letter from the General Board to the effect that '*your name has come to the top of the list for a college fellowship*' This was under some University statue no doubt dating back to the middle ages; it seemed to me to be rather an ungracious way of making such an offer. I felt that by that time I had managed very well with out one and a fellowship would no longer benefit me and I was by then too specialised in my work, to be of any use to the college or its students, I declined.

It must appear from this story that my relationship with the University was not of the best. Perhaps I was, and have remained, too much of a loner to fit well into the sort of academic camaraderie of college life. On the positive side the University allowed me to carry on with my chosen work unhindered and with out anytime consuming routine and with no commitment to teaching which was never my métier. They paid me regularly, if not always generously and, finally, they supplied me with a reasonable pension. However it did seem to me, at least as far as I was concerned,that they hardly lived up to Disraeli's standards.

CHAPTER 9

Looking Back

Apologia pro vita sua
John Henry Newman

Abstract: Looking back covers the highlights of my career. When I qualified as a doctor in 1945 medicine, by present day standards, was rather primitive with few effective therapies a good bedside manner was important. But there was little bureaucracy. Today it has changed out of all recognition as has the growth of bureaucratic control and meaningless Government targets The 1950s saw the start of this revolution in both new and highly effective drugs and high tech investigative techniques.. Two years in the army taught me little medicine but surely matured my outlook on life. On return to civilian medicine I learned about metabolic medicine and thanks to a year as a Fulbright fellow in the USA I was introduced to the problems of Wilson's disease which set the course for the rest of my life's work. This was continued with the development of effective therapies, in the environment of the University of Cambridge and at Addenbrooke's Hospital. On reaching retiring age I was able to continue work at University College Hospital and then the Middlesex Hospital in London until I took a well earned retirement at the age of 80 years.

Initially I considered entitling this last chapter 'Retrospectroscopy' but on further consideration I decided that this would be over the top and I settled for the more prosaic 'Looking Back'. Most of us, I suppose, must do this when we come to retire. I have said nothing about my years as a medical student in London except for the rather exciting story of a delivery during the time of the buzz bombs. I have been asked what about student parties ? Those who have not lied through out the black out, war time shortages and the necessity of passing exams at the first attempt can not realize why such activities were simply not on the agenda.. For myself looking back over almost 50 years work concentrated on a single rare disease it might, at first sight, seem a life rather ill spent. It is over 60 years since I first qualified in medicine in 1945 and medicine has changed out of all recognition in that time. There were very few effective drugs in the therapeutic armamentarium of those days, the sulphonamides for infection, morphia for pain, insulin for diabetes, crude extracts of the thyroid and adrenal glands for hormone deficiencies and liver extract for pernicious anaemia besides a collection of placebos which may, or may not have helped. Otherwise medicine was ineffective and a bedside manner, now surely a lost art, a thing of great importance. After qualification I held a six months appointment as house physician to the Professor of Medicine, Professor (later Sir Harold) Himsworth and then two years as a general duty medical officer in the Royal Army Medical Corps. During those two years I was posted to the Middle East theatre and I learned the importance of good hygiene and keeping a fully up to date inoculation status in my regiment but little of medicine despite two short spells in military hospital in Athens and Nicosia. I did learn of the quite breathless beauty of the Greek countryside before the dead hand of development and the tourist trade set about destroying this for ever. I also learned something of the problems of guerilla war in Palestine which reminds me of the story of the revolver. Having completed my tour of duty in Greece I was posted to a Field Dressing Station (FDS) on the coast in Palestine. I was flown, at short notice, in a Lancaster with other troops to Heliopolis south of Cairo thence I caught train to Haifa. That particular day a High Court judge was kidnapped from his court, I forget whether it was in Jerusalem or Tel Aviv, and this held up all movement for 24 hours. On reaching my unit I was issued with a revolver for my own protection and that of 'my patients'. I had never held a lethal weapon before and was given no instruction on its use. I duly carried this about with me by day and slept with it under my pillow, as commanded, by night. Not very comfortable. After about a week the entire unit was marched down to the beach for target practice. When first issued with the revolver I decided it would be much safer to load only five of the six chambers with bullets. Thus on reaching the beach I thought I had better pull

John Walshe (Ed.)

the trigger to get a bullet opposite the barrel before being commanded to aim and fire at the target. No one had told me that it was not the chamber opposite the barrel that was discharged on pulling the trigger (hence revolver) but the next one up. Thus when I withdrew my weapon from the holster and pulled the trigger I was shaken when it fired and a hole appeared in the beach next to my foot. I then realized the meaning of 'Shooting yourself in the foot'. I decided that I was not competent with such a dangerous toy and gave my revolver back to the Quarter Master forthwith. On my way home, for demobilization in April 1948, I watched Jews and Arabs fighting it out in the streets from the deck of a trooper in Haifa harbour.

After demobilization I returned to academic medicine with a post on the Medical Unit at University College Hospital and it was at this stage that I cam under the influence of Charles Dent and his work on metabolic disease. It was then that I started work on aminoacid metabolism and, so as to pursue this I applied for and was awarded The Stothert Research Fellowship of the Royal Society. Thus, apart from my year as a Fulbright scholar at the Boston City Hospital, I stayed on the Medical Unit at University College Hospital until I moved to Cambridge in 1957. I have often asked myself were those 45 years between 1955 and the year 2000 well spent concentrated as they were on a single rare inherited disease. I very much doubt if any hospital accountant would consider such an activity cost effective. I have managed to convince myself that they probably were and I feel sure my patients would agree. It is not as if only the three hundred or so patients I actually looked after in this period benefited from my work. Many hundred, perhaps thousands of patients all over the world, most of whom have never heard of me, have been saved from an untimely and very unpleasant death, as a direct result of my researches. It has been, I think I can reasonably conclude, time well spent and of which I can reasonably be proud. I need, therefore no *apologia*. I fear, however, that in the present attitude to medical research and the current views on cost effectiveness and the litigious culture which now prevails that it is a sequence of events which is most unlikely to be replicated. Sometimes I refer to myself as the last of the dinosaurs. That I have been lucky there is no doubt. It was a fortunate coincidence that I was working on the Medical Unit at UCH when Charles Dent was establishing the first metabolic unit in Britain and that he found a corner for me in his laboratory. I was lucky to be asked to investigate the first patient in Britain to undergo a liver resection for cancer. I was lucky that he was treated with penicillin post operatively. I was lucky to be asked to see a patient with Wilson disease whilst working in the liver unit at the Boston City Hospital and I was extremely lucky that Charles Davidson was able to get some penicillamine for me to try out my idea. Again I was lucky that there were no restrictions in force to prevent this type of highly speculative venture from being pursued. Finally I was lucky that circumstances permitted me to continue this line of research as a life's work. Certainly I was helped by a series of coincidences which are unlikely to recur. The present day career structure which a young doctor must follow to reach the top would seem to be too rigid to allow him to indulge in research; academic medicine is the choice of the few. I was lucky also to meet some exceptionally able colleagues working in this field who all proved most cooperative in sharing ideas There were also some controversies, for instance that with the Uzman/Denny Brown school being the most obvious.

Over and above the satisfaction of knowing that I was directly responsible for saving many lives and that none of the major hypotheses I had put forward had subsequently been proved wrong there were other advantages in this line of work. Medicine is now bedeviled with conferences, mostly huge international meetings which are little more than bean feasts and add little to the sum total of human knowledge. There is a brand of internationally established doctors who might be known as symposionauts who flit from conference to conference reporting the work of their juniors, they have no time to do any of their own On the other hand small specialist meeting of experts are of value. You meet other workers directly involved in the same line of research and can exchange new ideas on the cutting edge of research. These meetings also have the merit in that it is possible to decide, critically, whose work is really valuable and who is a 'me too' investigator. Wilson disease was the basis of regular such specialist meetings over the years. The first, convened by Professor Cumings and myself, was held at The National Hospital for Nervous Diseases in London in 1961. The feature of this meeting which most sticks in my mind was a furious letter I received from Uzman, in reply to an invitation to attend, refusing to come because, so he claimed, no one would support his hypothesis. What he should have done was to grasp the opportunity to state his case. It was rather like Achilles sulking in his tent.

Then there was the Tokyo meeting. I found that it was only a little more expensive to fly round the world than to go straight there and back. En route I took the opportunity to stop off in Athens and see some of my Greek patients and revisit the sites I had first seen when serving in the Royal Army Medical Corps in that theatre at the end of the war. Then on to a stop off in Delhi with a chance to see the Tomb of Akbar, the Red Fort and the Taj Mahal., a memorable experience. Tokyo itself I found very much like any other modern city. As for the conference I remember no epoch making contributions from delegates but one incident has stuck in my mind. A Japanese doctor said to me 'we have been reading your papers for such a long time now I thought you must be very old' As I was then in my mid forties I was not sure whether or not I should be flattered. After the meeting I joined with Herb Scheinberg and we visited the old imperial city of Kyoto. The journey in the Bullet train was quite an experience compared with British Rail. Unfortunately a passing hurricane deposited almost unmeasurable amounts of rain the day we visited the temples and moss gardens, I think I have never been so wet. After the meeting I flew back via Honoloulou. Passing the international date line I gained a day which I spent in that island, I had been booked into a rather disappointing little hotel by my travel agent, but it had the advantage of being close to Wakiki beach, but I regretted not having the chance to see other parts of the island. Thence I flew on to San Francisco and, after a short stay to Salt Lake City where I took the opportunity to visit Dr Cartwright, one of the pioneers of copper research, but who never attended conferences so he was, and remained somewhat elusive. Thence I tried to visit the Grand Canyon, but again appalling weather trumped by plans so I visited Santa Fe and Phoenix instead. My next eastwards flight took me over the Arizona desert, site of the first atomic explosion, before reaching New York and thence home.

There were other meetings, one in Norway in which I reported some studies I had done to disprove a theory that there were abnormalities of copper metabolism in patients with schizophrenia. This was sponsored by NATO, though what their interest this organization could possible have in copper metabolism I can not even guess. The next meeting of which I have a lasting memory was at Pilsen at which I was able to report basic studies on the metabolism of radiolabelled trientine. En route I met up with Herb Scheinberg and we had a few days exploring the beauties of Prague which, at that time was still behind the Iron Curtain. The official rate of exchange for the Pound against the Krona was very unfavourable but the hotel receptionist gave us a telephone number to ring for a better rate. Herb was all in favour of ringing this but I felt that, for all we knew, it might be a line straight to the secret police. However we found a satisfactory way of conducting this business, a short taxi ride round the town centre and the taxi driver gave us a rate of exchange three times the official one. We made several short taxi rides during our stay in the beautiful city. Another eastern European visit was to Warsaw and the last of my international conferences was to Leipzig, the programme here was so dense that there was no time for sight seeing. There were also three visits to Germany, the first as a guest lecturer to Bonn. Having a morning to spare I took the opportunity to visit Cologne and photograph the fourteenth century glass in the cathedral which had been saved from the ravages of wartime bombing. The next, a similar visit, was to Munich and this gave me the chance to see the wonderful eleventh century glass in Augsburg cathedral only a short train journey away. As my official contribution to this meeting had only been to talk at a 'working breakfast' I felt this made the visit worth while. Finally I was invited to lecture in Berlin. I found it a trifle embarrassing that I spoke in English to an audience of German doctors who all clearly understood and their questions to me afterwards, in perfect English, proved this point. I seriously felt my lack of a foreign language was a real handicap. I apologized to my audience explaining that, long ago when I was at school, a knowledge of Latin and Greek was considered of more importance than modern languages. As Ann my wife was unable to travel by air, she had suffered serious trouble with her ears on a flight to join me in New York in the early 1960s, it meant that she missed out on all this foreign visits. However there were two conference to which she was able to come; \an early one in Paris and another, again sponsored by NATO, on this occasion the subject was 'Orphan Drugs' This was held in Brussels. We took the opportunity to visit Bruges en route and relive a happy stay there way back in the 1950s. For Ann it was but a poor return for the many times I had, perforce, left her at home.

One extracurricular activity gave me particular pleasure. In 1989 a very old friend, Dr James Fisher, rang me to say that there was some interesting stained glass in a private school near Bournemouth, to which he was medical officer. He invited me to stay and see the glass. I readily accepted and was delighted to see, in the front hall of the school, the former seat of the Earls of Malmsbury, four large panels of continental glass probably from a Jesse window. Research soon showed me that this glass was quite unknown and unrecorded. I immediately informed English Heritage and made considerable efforts, unfortunately unsuccessful, to determine the original home of the glass and the time of its translation to this country. I was eventually able published this finding some 18 years later.

The passing of the years inevitably brought it's sadnesses. The first half of the year 2009 signaled the loss of three friends and colleagues. The first to depart this mortal coil was Irmin Sternlieb, perhaps the junior figure in the Scheinberg-Sternlieb partnership, based at the Albert Einstein College of medicine in New York City. Apart from being a fine gastroenterologist he was a magnificent linguist and, together with Scheinberg was in charge of perhaps the largest number of patients with Wilson disease in any clinic. A few months later I learned of the death of Herb Scheinberg, a great friend and most helpful colleague over more than 50 years, this was a great sadness. Finally Alick Bearn also died. In the late 1950s he had given me hospitality in his laboratory at the Rockefeller Institute, later University, and allowed me to make some observation on his patients at a time when my own clinic was too small to carry out such studies. He also kindly arranged for me to stay, cost free, in the VIP suite at the Institute and Ann, my wife, was able to join me there for part of my stay. This was a great help in getting my own line of research established.

Before I close I would like to relate my thoughts on committee work. When I first joined the consultant staff at the old Addenbrooke's Hospital I found that I had a place, as of right, on the consultant staff committee meetings In those days the staff was relatively small and to attend these meetings was an opportunity to get to know my new colleagues, also to see how the hospital was run; before the wave of bureaucratization that has swept through the Health Service in recent years, the consultant staff did have a real voice in deciding policy. It also had the advantage that an excellent tea was supplied at the meeting. The efficiency of these committees varied very much with the chairman. The first I encountered ran the meetings with great efficiency, he made all the decisions and the committee members were little more than ciphers. The second chairman was quite incapable of controlling a meeting and these wandered on aimlessly to no useful purpose. The third chairman was ideal, he could control a meeting whilst allowing sensible discussion of difficult points. I soon discovered that if one spoke up there was a grave risk of being appointed to a sub committee to discuss the point in question and come up with a report so I learned to observe in silence. The second thing I learned was that the only firm decision ever made at these big committees was the date of the next meeting, all other decisions were deferred to the relevant sub committees. This had the additional advantage for the chairman was that he could not be held responsible for any mistaken decisions. He could always say that perforce he acted on the advice of his expert subcommittee. Eventually I decided that time spent on committee work was wasted and I would do better to carry on work in my laboratory.

Later, when I was promoted to the post of Reader in Metabolic Disease, I found myself, ex officio, on the degree committee of the Faculty Board of Medicine, that was for the award of higher degrees, doctors of philosophy and doctors of medicine. Before I attended my first meeting I was taken aside by one of the senior members and told that I really must attend to try and prevent professor A and B from siphoning through doubtful candidates! Again we never had to make any hard decisions, The degree of PhD was awarded for a thesis written after a three years research project carried out under supervision, and the MD, either for a thesis or for published work. All the committee did was to appoint referees to consider the work and report back. In the event of the referees disagreeing we then appointed a third one to adjudicate. Now arose one of those decisions by the University, the logic of which eluded me. The Regius Professor decided that the medical degree committee should be able to award the degree of doctor of science, ScD., hitherto this degree was in the gift of the faculty of Biology B, to whom I had submitted my own published work some years earlier. At that time it was considered to be one of the most difficult of the degrees to achieve. Why the medical degree committee should award the ScD I found difficult to understand. However the General Board of the Faculties conceded to the Regius' wish and we were hence forth able to award this degree. I wondered what would have happened if Biology B had petitioned to award he degree of MD. It seemed to me that what ever decision the General Board had made to such a request would be inherently illogical. Such is the wisdom of 600 years accumulated in an ancient seat of learning, who was I to question it? Being a cynic* I have come to the conclusion that Pontius Pilate should be appointed patron saint of committees and that his portrait, washing his hands, should hang in all committee rooms. This might bring home to the chairman that offloading responsibility does not necessarily give the correct decision.

Following my final retirement in the year 2000 I have endeavoured to keep in touch with my old patients and have supported and regularly attended the meetings of the Wilson's Disease Support Group besides writing the occasional article for their journal and continuing to write articles for scientific journals summarizing previously unpublished results of my researches. I have also been pleased to supply advice to patients and their relatives, either on the telephone or by e-mail when so requested but it really looks as if the last drop of perspiration, that followed the moment of inspiration, has been shed. I am tempted to end with the words of the poet,

When men of science find out something more
We shall be happier then we were before

Unfortunately the story does not have a happy ending. There was to come one final sting in the tail. This was the decision of the General Medical Councils to remove from the medical register all over age doctors. I felt this was hardly a just reward for a life spent on the improvement in medical practice to which I had contributed so much. To add insult to injury was the somewhat threatening tone of the letter which informed me, and presumably many colleagues, of this decision. It fell below the standard of courtesy one could reasonably expect from such a 'distinguished' body.

* I would like to define a cynic as a failed pessimist.

INDEX